THE PSYCHEDELIC BIBLE

EVERYTHING YOU NEED TO KNOW ABOUT
PSILOCYBIN MAGIC MUSHROOMS, 5-MEO
DMT, LSD / ACID & MDMA

ALEX GIBBONS

Copyright © 2019 Alex Gibbons.

All rights reserved. No part of this publication may be reproduced, distributed or transmitted in any form or by any means, including photocopying, recording, or other electronic or mechanical methods, without the prior written permission of the publisher, except in the case of brief quotations embodied in critical reviews and certain other non-commercial uses permitted by copyright law.

Trademarked names appear throughout this book. Rather than use a trademark symbol with every occurrence of a trademarked name, names are used in an editorial fashion, with no intention of infringement of the respective owner's trademark. The information in this book is distributed on an "as is" basis, without warranty. Although every precaution has been taken in the preparation of this work, neither the author nor the publisher shall have any liability to any person or entity with respect to any loss or damage caused or alleged to be caused directly or indirectly by the information contained in this book.

UPDATES

For a chance to go into the draw to win a FREE book every month like our 'Stoner Themed Coloring Book' (below), and other updates on our latest books, subscribe below!

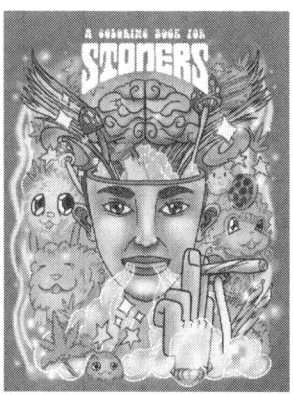

https://psychedeliccuriosity.activehosted.com/f/1

For daily posts on all things Psychedelic, follow us on Instagram @Psychedelic.curiosity

Psychedelics are illegal not because a loving government is concerned that you may jump out of a third story window. Psychedelics are illegal because they dissolve opinion structures and culturally laid down models of behaviour and information processing. They open you up to the possibility that everything you know is wrong.

— Terrence McKenna

PART I

AN INTRODUCTORY GUIDE TO MAGIC MUSHROOMS

THE BEGINNERS PSYCHEDELIC EXPLORER'S GUIDE OF THIS HALLUCINOGENIC PLANT

Mushrooms can heal, feed and possibly enlighten you - maybe even help save the world.

— Dr. Paul Stamets

1
INTRODUCTION

Nature's psychedelic truffles, magic mushrooms, have been part of human cultures for thousands of years. From the Sahara to Guatemala, they have always provided human beings with a natural means to get high. What's more, they have been part of arts and culture, as well as academic interest, and have held great ritual and spiritual importance in cultures across the globe.

'Shrooms', or magic mushrooms, are what we call the fungi that have hallucinogenic properties called psilocybin. They are naturally growing psychedelic drugs with a long history and an intertwined relationship with human cultures across the globe. They produce mind-altering effects and cause hallucinations, out-of-the-ordinary thought patterns and hypnotic and trance-like states. The experiences encountered on magic mushrooms are generally called a 'trip.'

They grow in the wild in woodlands, grasslands and plains and are fairly universal in their distribution. They can also be cultivated artificially but they are illegal in many countries. The fascinating thing is, they have long been taken for recreational use, healing functions and in spiritual and creative endeavors. They were rediscovered in the west in the 1950s, and remain one of the most popular hallucinogens in under 35s in the United States according to some reports.

We have written this beginner's guide to take you on a journey through the fun, the facts, the science, the dangers and the benefits of magic mushrooms. While reading this won't qualify you as a *mycologist* - a mushroom expert - or instantly make you a mushroom guru like Stamet - a world-leading mycologist - it will offer you everything you need to know to begin your journey of discovery about magic mushrooms, types, history, culture, dosage, trips (historical and modern day), side effects, dangers, scientific research, and much more. While we don't advocate their use, growth or illegal activity in any way, we are offering you everything we know and have found about magic mushrooms in order for you to remain aware.

Through this explorer's guide, you will see through case reports, or 'trip' reports, academic research and historical records of magic mushrooms on cave paintings. These mystical little fungi have sparked emotions and experiences as diverse as the spectrum of the entire universe. From euphoria, visual alterations, right through to creative impulses, paranoia or anxiety, they have played a significant role in the human experience throughout time and across space.

Beginning our guide, you can go on a journey through time and space through the prism of magic mushrooms in the section about history and culture.

We then explore the most common types of magic mushrooms, and look at their active properties. This section describes the physical features of the two most common types and how to identify them, as well as the dangers of picking magic mushrooms. We explore some little-known stories and look at the first ever trip report from 1799, and the first viral trip report from 1955 that let a huge mushroom-shaped, Mexican secret, out of the bag for good.

We then shift a gear to look at the recreational use of magic mushrooms. If you are interested in the ways people get hold of magic mushrooms, or grow them, you can explore those themes and also look at dosages, the longevity and preparation of magic mushrooms, and how they are ingested.

Do you want to know what it is like to experience magic mushrooms without taking them? Don't take your friends' word for it, or look at the mystical depictions in films. We avoid glamourising mushrooms and give you an array of real-life experiences from real life trip reports; the next best thing to experiencing them yourself. We summarise three experiences found by journalers online which all give genuine insights into the inner world of magic mushrooms from different perspectives. These are the good, the bad, the ugly, and everything in between. Get a clearer picture of the array of emotions that happen while on a magical mushroom journey. What's more, these experiences are all backed by cases within scientific research. You may even begin to see patterns emerging; psychedelic ones.

We outline the dangers of magic mushrooms and point out what is going on at a chemical level in the brain too. Following this, we offer up a few findings from recent studies on psychedelic therapies and the potential for possible benefits to mental health disorders outlined by a few scholars.

If you want a quick fact sheet, we provide a FAQs section at the end; a speedy glance at everything you might need to know about magic mushrooms, simply put. As a bonus, we give you some quick-fire do's and don'ts. As with everything in this guide, as we tell you in the legalities section, mushrooms are illegal. We just want you to have the facts and know what to do to keep as safe as possible, or stop you or your tripping friends from going into a hole.

So, sit back, relax, and enjoy this explorer's guide…

2

HISTORY

Magic mushrooms came back to Europe in the 1950s when a *mycologist* called Wisson traveled through Mexico to study them. A huge stir came about; this man published his findings in *Life* magazine, and people began to flock to the drug. There was an outcry from governments, and these were just the thing young hippies had been looking for to make a break from the previous generation. This article is in no small part one of the things that sparked the psychedelic era: a wave of popular culture and a whole movement was fuelled somewhat by the recreational use of magic mushrooms. What most people don't know, however, is that 'shrooms' date back to way before, into ancient times. People were recording trip reports before the invention of writing.

Deep into the caves of the baking hot Sahara desert, there are depictions of magic mushrooms that have been dated to 9000 BC in what is now Algeria. Early hunter-gatherers painted on cave walls, leaving us a record of their experiences of magic mushrooms. Historians are convinced these are *Psilocybe Mairei*, a local mushroom of the area. It seems the properties of mushrooms in opening up different avenues of the mind have meant they were used in spiritual contexts. Who knows, some of these experiences may have been profound, godly and spiritual, and some may have led to introspective staring at the infinite grains of sand on the desert! We can imagine that humans have always experienced the natural psychoactive properties of mushrooms in ways that are unique to them as a person, yet profoundly human and universal.

And in Europe? Spotted in Spain, there was a real buzz some years ago when a research team discovered 6000-year-old rock art on a cave mural. The Selva Pascuala mural is just outside the town of Villar del Humo and is the oldest evidence of their use in Europe.

This painting mainly depicts a bull but also interestingly shows thirteen small little capped mushrooms along the bottom of the painting. Due to their long, fine, stems, varying between straight and curvy, and their small dome-like caps, just like the real thing, the famous expert in Psilocybe, Gaston Guzman, confirmed that these are local versions of the mushrooms with hallucinogenic properties called *Psilocybe hispanica*.[1]

It is likely, therefore, these were used to open up new perspectives and cognitive experiences, perhaps during religious rituals, or even during artistic expression itself.

The spiritual

While their use may have oscillated between recreational and spiritual over time, the transcendent properties endowed to humans by mushrooms mean that they have often been utilized in ceremonial practices, shamanic rituals and by spirit mediums, as well as those on a more personal spiritual journey.

Where these cave paintings occurred in areas that mushrooms grow, there is some artistic proof that hallucinogenic mushrooms were used in controlled ritual practices with numerous dimensions and strands. On these rock paintings were portrayals of god-like figures wearing masks and adorned with mushrooms, where ritual offerings were made.

Coupled with evidence from other parts of the world, it is thought that magic mushrooms were taken with great ritual importance, in events of mystic-religious practices. Ancient Mayan and Aztec peoples were thought to use magic mushrooms to produce trance-like states, communicate with gods, and create visions.[2] Not much unlike modern-day experiences, as you can check out in the trip reports and recorded stories later in this guide.

The psyche

Shrooms spiraling out of human heads, tripping, painting and describing. These depictions were left in the far reaches of the Artic many years ago. While this was way before sharing and 'going viral', depictions of *the effects* of magic mushrooms were left in another old-school record. Scholar, Dikov, discovered the Pegtymel petroglyph 40 miles (60 kilometers) from the Arctic on the Pegtymel River, with funky pictures of people with mushrooms coming out of their heads, reminiscent of psychedelic art.[3]

Could these be an early artist's way of showing the effects that mushrooms have on the human psyche? This particular strain was thought to be *Amanita* Mushrooms, or *Amanita Muscaria*, ingested by the Chukchi people.

A creative impulse

One thread running through this guide, and it seems over time, is the creative impulse that comes about through magic mushrooms. Just like in the psychedelic sixties there is an idea that hallucinogens have provided inspiration for artistic depictions themselves, or that these early artists were under the influence of magic mushrooms.

Lewis-Williams and Dowson, in 1988, put forward that there are many cave depictions or petroglyphs that were painted under the influence of mind-altering natural produce. European petroglyphs are covered in non-literal images and patterns such as lines, zigzags and circles, all thought to be potentially produced when in a mind-altered state.

This creative buzz is something that can be carried through to the psychedelic era right into the modern day. We will see a bit of this creative impulse further on in trip report one, a doodler from the U.S. who documents his experiences in drawings and writings.

Mushrooms in the psychedelic sixties: Psychedelic art and music

In Europe and the States, throughout the psychedelic sixties and seventies, mushrooms took people on new spiritual journeys that became characteristic of the era, along with their synthetic friend, LSD, or acid. Psychedelia characterized the day and made up a whole subculture that would carry on through decades of music, art and popular influence.

Like the thought process while on magic mushrooms, this art was hypnotic, varied in patterns and mystical. Bright colors and dissonant, deep, distorted, trippy, sounds, permeated the human psyche, where youth movements, free-living and a move towards open-mindedness provided a counter-culture to the backdrop of the post-war decades. Think late Beatles, think sitar, think Sergeant Pepper's.

Once more, experiences on mind-altering drugs were depicted in art, which used vibrant colors, non-representational forms, shapes and spectrums to try to recreate the experiences encountered whilst tripping. This art and music not only artistically reflects the tripping journey, it was created to be enjoyed whilst experiencing the effects of mushrooms themselves.

Our next section takes a little look at what magic mushrooms are, and the facts. We do go into some more early experiences in this section, before looking at the recreational side of the drugs and trip reports.

3
WHAT'S IN A 'SHROOM'? THE FACTS

These natural growing hallucinogens have played a part in culture at various moments in history, but what exactly are they? And what is in them to induce some of the feelings we have talked about already?

What are magic mushrooms?

Magic mushrooms are small fungal species that contain the properties that trigger certain neurochemical responses in the brain. There are hundreds upon hundreds of types of psilocybin-containing species growing all over the world. We might call them magic little fungal globetrotters.

So, what's in them?

The hallucinogenic substances within the mushroom are psilocybin, psilocin and baeocystin, known to induce various effects on the human brain, such as euphoria, altered consciousness, dissolving of the ego (sense-of-self), altered behavior and concentration span, anxiety and paranoia. In fact, there is a whole array of responses and magic mushroom experiences that depend on the person, the environment, and the dose.

Neurochemical effects: what it does to the brain

Scientists have a pretty good idea about the chemical ways mushrooms affect the brain. Psilocybin binds to the 5-HT2A receptor, the serotonin receptor in the brain, thus sparking a wave of electrochemical signals.[4]

The chemical makeup of psilocybin, psilocin and serotonin are actually pretty similar, as represented in the following visual (figure 1). Psilocin hence attaches itself to serotonin, which is the brain's chemical way of making us happy.

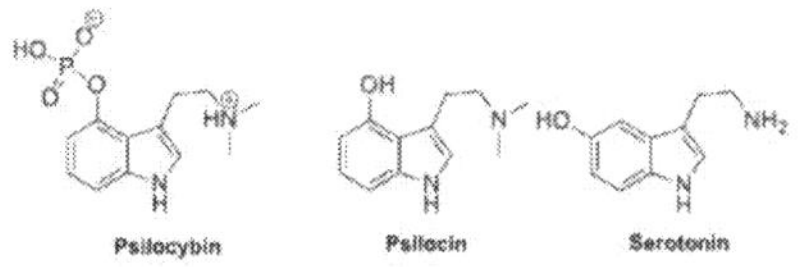

Figure 1. The structures of the main components of Psilocybe, psilocybin and psilocin, show marked similarity with serotonin.

If you are listening to the audio see the attached pdf guide to look at the images.

The legality of magic mushrooms

The schedule 1 drugs psilocin and psilocybin mean that possession of the mushrooms containing them in the United States is illegal. Spores do not contain these substances but are nonetheless illegal in Georgia, Idaho and California. However, selling spores is illegal in all states, especially selling them for the purposes of growing hallucinogenic mushrooms: it is outlawed by the Louisiana State Act 1959.

There have been some moves to legalize magic mushrooms, by those jumping on the cannabis bandwagon. A few in Denver and Oregon, for example, are pushing for its decriminalization. They are using the potential scientific research into the controlled use of psychedelics in treating mental health disorders as their springboard for this action.

Interesting fact: mushrooms were legal in the UK until very recently. Until 2005, you could pop to your local market or head shop and buy them over the counter and at music festivals. 'Shroom' dealers could have business cards and display posters of the various types: 'Harry Potters' and 'Mexican Blues', displaying pictures on their walls. Oddly, they went straight from 'legal' to class A, the most serious category of illegal drugs (along with heroin and cocaine) in the UK. Rumour has it that they became illegal during a few music festivals in August, where mushroom vendors had to give them away after midnight when the law changed and they could no longer sell them.

What types are there?

There are way too many types of psilocybin mushrooms to list in total here, over 180. There are books dedicated to the topic. The foremost expert is Stamets, but our further reading section gives you some insight into the books available. That said, let's have a look at some common types, and a few bonus 'shrooms' thrown in there for your interest. Most of them have pretty long Latin names but, of course, as anyone who has bought mushrooms would tell you, they have a whole host of street names, strains and types too.

We'll start off with one of the most commonly known, Liberty Caps, or *Psilocybe Semilanceata*.

Liberty Caps

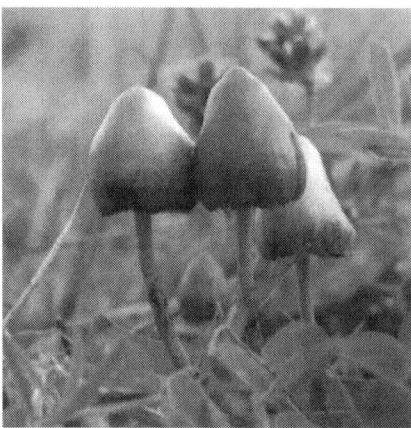

Figure 2. Fruit bodies of the hallucinogenic mushroom Psilocybe Semilanceata. Specimens photographed in Sweden.

This little shroom really packs a punch as one of the most potent around. It grows nearly everywhere there are wet grasslands: from the UK and Austria, to the Channel Islands, the Pacific Northwest and British Columbia. There are a few reports of its presence in the hill regions of Tamil Nadu in India. Figure 2 shows you Liberty Caps in *situ* in Sweden, quite innocent looking, right?

Five ways to identify Liberty Caps

While we strongly advise against picking your own mushrooms (in fact, this is the greatest danger attached to the drug and can result in death), there are 5 ways you can identify Liberty Caps for scientific purposes:

1. Firstly, think about where they are found and what type of

terrain (grassy wetlands in Europe and parts of North America and Canada).
2. Secondly, look at the cap of the mushroom itself to see if it is small and conical.
3. Number three sounds obvious, but observe carefully the color and the size and shape of the stem, which should be lighter than the brown cap, long and thin.
4. Next, check out the gills (the bits underneath the cap). You should see that the gills are narrowly attached and cream in color.
5. Final top tip: to be 100% sure, you can take a spore print by leaving it on a piece of paper for 2-6 hours. You can then look under a microscope.

Liberty Caps can be found growing in autumn mostly, before the first frosts, and normally in September. Seasoned 'shroomers' live for this picking season, and their annual trip to a known spot. As our legal section outlines, possession of any form of magic mushrooms is against the law in most countries. Not only that, they are very easily misidentified.

Liberty Caps have a pretty interesting case study from London we wanted to share with you. We could call this the first written trip report in history.

The first trip report in history: A family affair

So unlike other trip reports in this guide, this one was not found online. It wasn't your typical spiritual journey or even an expected trip to begin with. It happened in 1799 in London, with a man and his kids. This trip was a bit of a family affair and is one of the first modern documented uses of Liberty Caps and of mushrooms in Europe. [5]

Imagine this, you, your mum, and your dad, munch upon an innocent looking mushroom in the park before you all temporarily lose your minds, burst into fits of laughter and total and utter confusion, and watch each other's pupils dilate. This is what happened to a father of four in 1799 when he made a family meal with mushrooms picked in London's Green Park. This is not only an interesting bit of history, it gives you some insight into the effects of magic mushrooms. It also gives a 'family day trip' a whole new meaning.

Trip report disclaimers and warnings

This story could be one of those urban myths! It should be noted that in general, overcooking mushrooms takes away their psychoactive properties. So unless this guy made a mushroom salad, there could be some slight exaggeration involved here. Still, it is a 'charming' story, aside from the thought of child abuse! Obviously, it goes without saying that giving children any substances, illicit or otherwise, is completely and utterly abhorrent, even in 1799.

Since 1998, Liberty Caps come with a bit of an additional warning label too: there have been reports of traces of phenethylamine in them, which could cause adverse reactions. Scientists are not too sure about the exact amounts of the phenethylamine within them yet, but it is well worth noting that anything growing and illegal is unregulated and untested, and thus a bit of a lottery.

The next mushroom on our list has its roots in Mexico...

4
THE MEXICAN: PSILOCYBE CUBENSIS

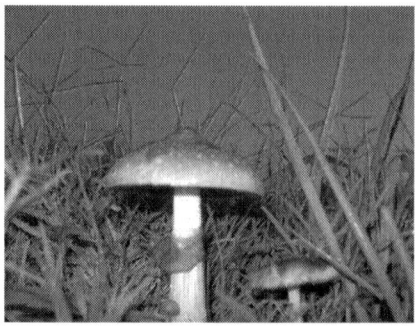

Figure 3. Psilocybe Cubensis. Source: WikiCommons. Credit: Rohan523 (2009).

Another mushroom commonly found is the *Psilocybe Cubensis*. This one has a tall thick stalk in comparison to the Liberty Cap. The middle of the stem is a bright blue, indicating potent amounts of the substance psilocin. This gives them a pretty psychedelic appearance on the inside, despite their innocent looking exterior. The picture of the dried mushrooms in figure 4 shows their bluish tinge.

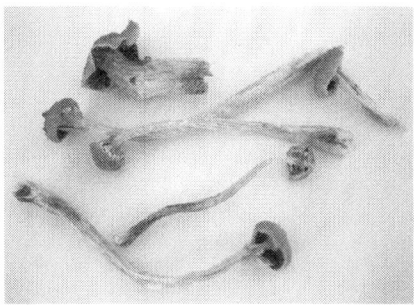

Figure 4. Dried Psilocybe Cubensis magic mushrooms. Source: wiki commons. Credit: Erik Fenderson (2006).

In the Netherlands, where there are some slightly more relaxed laws on magic mushrooms, this mushroom is called a Mexican mushroom because, you guessed it, this mushroom is largely found in Mexico. This psychedelic is an extremely popular natural psychedelic drug.

It is readily found as it is easy to grow. In Holland, while the mushroom itself is banned, you can by grow kits well within the limits of the law. Figure 5 shows these cubensis growing in a box at home and figure 6 shows the magnified spore print. Spore prints are a bit like the fingerprint of a mushroom, and each one has its own unique pattern when observed under a microscope.

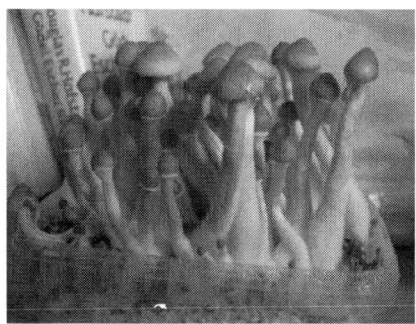

Figure 5. Growbox with nearly mature p. Cubensis. Source: WikiCommons. Credit: LordToran

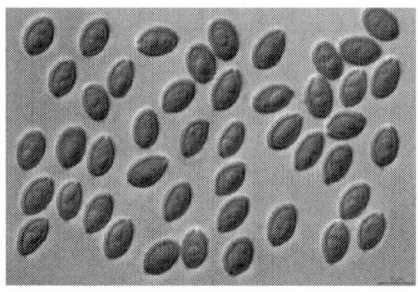

Figure 6. Psilocybe Cubensis spores, 1000 times magnification illuminated with DIC. Source: Wikicommons, Alan Rockefella (2013).

A 1950s trip report that went 'viral'

The Mexican secret of thousands of years was let out the bag by a curious American researcher in the 1950s. The Velada, Maria Sabina and the 'healing' Mexican mushroom became a smash hit around the world.

This Mexican mushroom was encountered by a mushroom expert through the ritual session of a certain Maria Sabina. The secret was let out the bag, causing a wave of trippers, both physically and metaphorically, to flock to the Mexican (the person and the mushroom).[6]

In Mexico, the *Psilocybe Cubensis* mushroom had been used in the Velada session for centuries. Maria Sabina used mushrooms to communicate with the gods and heal the sick in this ritualistic practice.

In the early 1950s, Wasson met the Mazatec curandera (medicine woman or healer) Maria Sabina, before eating mushrooms and recording them, sending a craze around the world for these psychedelic drugs. While this practice had largely been a secret for the rest of the world and carried out by experienced practitioners in Mexico, this was the start of recreational discovery. News of this mushroom went wild, and the *Psilocybe Cubensis* had more than its fifteen minutes of fame. Hippie tourists flocked to Maria's village for a hit, and the Mexican mushroom was used far and wide in the United States until it was banned in 1966. The banning of this mushroom in Mexico in 1970 saw the total end of this practice but not of the mushroom, which is still sold illegally, and grown. So, this 'trip report' wasn't shared online either but certainly had a monumental impact, introducing the world of mushrooms, tripping, and psychedelics, to a vast audience.[7]

Psilocybe azurescens, or 'Azzies'

These are reportedly the most potent of all mushrooms, containing massive amounts of psychoactive compounds that make you trip. It bruises blue, demonstrating the high levels of psilocin. This one also contains baeocystin and norbaeocystin and is reportedly capable of paralyzing your muscles.

It is found, but only by absolute experts (who keep their location secret) in the Pacific Northwest U.S. People have been known to buy the spores online and have encountered a few batches (probably through amateur growth outdoors). As usual, the mushroom guru, Stamets, reported its discovery back in 1995.

A highbrow trip report, from a professional writer

Writers do have a way with words, something that is equally useful and misleading at times. Michael Pollan paints a somewhat pretty picture of his experiences on 'azzies', which he picked with Stamets himself of all people. Not only did he write a compelling book, *How to Change Your Mind: What the New Science of Psychedelics Teaches Us About Consciousness, Dying, Addiction, Depression, and Transcendence*, he published an engaging extract online, in the Atlantic, no less.

He pitches some pretty interesting questions to academics about why, biologically, ecologically, and from an evolutionary perspective, mushrooms contain psychoactive properties. "Was it a defense mechanism to ward-off being eaten? And, how are the spores dispersed?", he asked. The answers lead to a mention of some pretty out-there animal trip reports. Horses getting high. Whatever next? His own, artsy, well-crafted, trip report is worth a read, but these mushrooms are probably best avoided by your average Joe.

5
THE RECREATIONAL USE OF MUSHROOMS

Aside from the facts, the history and the scientific info, we come right into the recreational use of mushrooms. If they are illegal, where do people get them? What do they do with them when they do? And how do they experience them?

Where do you get magic mushrooms?

While shrooms can be found growing in most countries around the world, most people avoid hunting and picking them themselves. Not least because possession of them is illegal in most countries because of the banned substances within them but, moreover, because there are so many varieties of mushrooms.

Even in a best-case scenario where you don't pick a toxic mushroom, you won't trip because picking a similar looking strain of the cousin you are after won't contain psilocybin. A slightly better (but not so brilliant) outcome of picking the wrong mushrooms would be a dodgy stomach, severe cramps or even hospitalization.

Most people will tell you, picking a mushroom with only a slightly different diameter cap could result in death. The big laughing gym, as it is commonly referred, will do a bit of both: it has psilocybin (probably not even enough to get you high) but is classed as poisonous, making you sick and ripping your stomach to shreds.

Although they are illegal in most countries, there is always a black market for them. Mushrooms are generally sold in the U.S. in eighths, meaning one-eighth of an ounce (3.5 grams), which usually costs around $20.

Picking them wild is an option for some but, as we made clear above, it's a risk you don't want to take as identifying mushrooms can be difficult. Some people grow them at home, most commonly grown being *Cubensis*, as they are reportedly the easiest to grow.

In the UK, although the active component Psilocybe is illegal, whether sold dried, fresh or prepared, head shops get around this law by selling spores in suspension under the guise of being for microscopy and microbiological purposes.

People buy them in the form of spore syringes, costing between ten and twenty dollars in the U.S. You can buy spore prints which have to be rehydrated before growing. Information on how to grow can also be found in various places online. Again, this can be extremely tricky. Failing to create the kind of sterile environment mushrooms need to grow could result in contamination. Contamination can result in either unsuccessful crops or, worse still, a batch that is bad for you.

How much do you take?

Dosage is a lottery with shrooms. Beginners are advised to start on a low dose (one gram) because of the unknown effects of the mushrooms but also the very variable potencies of mushrooms. It is always worth waiting an hour to see how you feel at that point, although the experience will change over the course of the trip. The way the mushrooms are prepared can also cause issues. Different strains also have different effects and are advised in varying amounts. Likewise, whether the mushrooms are dried or fresh affects the dosage. *Cubensis* comes in various forms and its Thai versions, for example, are thought to be way stronger and more intense than the supposedly more mellow versions from the Gulf Coast.

Psilocybin is one of the main active properties of magic mushrooms and to feel the effects of the drug, you have to take between three and thirty mg. There is a bit more detail in our FAQ. People vary their doses from micro-dosing, to strong doses of up to five grams. Your tolerance to mushrooms decreases over time so people can find themselves having to take more and more in order to feel the same effects.

Micro-dosing is something that is said to induce creativity, while you won't feel the strong effects of mushrooms. Increasing the dose up to one gram may alter your perceptions slightly but would normally not cause changes to vision and states that medium strong doses of three grams and strong doses of five grams would.

How do people take magic mushrooms?

Mushrooms can be eaten fresh or dried, brewed into mushroom tea, taken in pill or liquid form, or prepared into other drinks or food.

Eating them

While it is possible to eat them, mushrooms are reported to have a terrible taste; either bitter or floury and are sort of saliva-inducing in a bad way. Eating fresh can also induce stomach cramps.

People have been known to come up with some funky ways to disguise the taste. You could cook a chilli, maybe even a mushroom pizza or a smoothie. Alternatively, for those non-cooks, peanut butter, jam, or fruit is another alternative. Or, some just have a drink at hand to wash them down. However, cooking the mushrooms too much with too much heat will give a weaker effect and reduce the impact of the psychoactive ingredient, psilocybin.

. . .

Mushroom tea and other drinks

Another popular alternative is mushroom tea. Be under no illusions, this is not your normal brew and may not taste or look particularly pleasant either.

Many people prefer to make mushroom tea rather than eat them fresh, which can lessen the effect of stomach upset but also make you feel the effects much more quickly. Stomach cramps can be really distracting and unwelcoming, especially if you are tripping for the first time.

Mushrooms can be cut into smaller bits, or for smaller varieties, you can boil them whole and make 'shroom tea'. The way to make tea is to brew the mushrooms for twenty minutes in hot water, leaving the fresh mushrooms at the bottom. The mushroom liquid (which could be a brownish color) is then poured into cups, and whole mushrooms or pieces are added to the cups too. These pieces of mushrooms can still be eaten after drinking the liquid itself but they won't be as strong. Tea will make you feel the effects more quickly but you will come down quicker as well.

Some people soak mushrooms in alcohol, such as tequila, and combine the two substances. In our mixology section, however, we do advise against such mixing.

Mushroom pills

Mushrooms could be ground and packed into gelatine pills. The taste and texture can be avoided this way, but it would be difficult to see what was inside each pill. You would not actually know what you are getting.

Mushroom mixology: drugs to avoid on magic mushrooms

Like all substances, things can mix around in your body in mysterious ways. We go into some detail here about what to avoid whilst taking magic mushrooms.

Mushrooms are generally considered fairly safe in comparison to some drugs in terms of pharmaceutical risks, however, when mixing, it can sometimes have negative reactions.

- **Tramadol/Prozac**

Because magic mushrooms are a serotonin agonist, it is not generally advised to take mushrooms whilst on these drugs. You will read varying reports online but there is limited scientific research. People with issues with mental health are generally to steer clear of mushrooms and other non-prescription drugs.

- **Cocaine /Amphetamines**

This mix is generally agreed on through experience and through scientific reports. Coke, LSD and mushrooms do not mix well on a chemical level or in terms of psychological effects. Reports go from "overpowers the trip" to "uncomfortable and edgy" and many people agree that coming down on coke is not fun whilst on mushrooms. As one "seasoned tripper" put it, they are on different ends of the "trip spectrum."

- **Alcohol**

Generally, alcohol will just make you more out of your senses and you won't experience the mushrooms in the same way. You may not notice the negative side effects of one which is a plus however, the alcohol could potentially make you sick.

6
THE EXPERIENCE

Now we are getting into the experiences of magic mushrooms, looking first of all at how it can change your sense-of-self and everything you know for a few short hours.

The effects take about half an hour, to an hour, to kick in, and they last for between five and seven hours. Some people enjoy psychedelic art surrounding them in the background, appreciate nice music, and some people like to just sit and chat, stare, reflect or share the experience together.

Some people record their experiences, writing or drawing things that come to mind, as the effects of psychedelic drugs have been known to induce creativity. You can read about peoples tripping journeys online.

Mushrooms are mind-altering, so people generally report on the importance of tripping in a safe environment. One key element from trip reports people post online is being around people you trust and avoiding situations where they need to make important decisions.

. . .

Losing yourself for a bit?

Ever heard of an out-of-body experience? Or felt a detachment from your sense of self, or like you were floating above your own body? At times, as humans, we can experience a sort of 'epiphany moment' when we suddenly see things outside of normal realms; behaviors and the feelings which dictate our actions can suddenly transform and we see things in a new way. What can happen with magic mushrooms is that they form temporary new connections between brain cells, making your brain function in different ways. Your thinking can be out of the ordinary, and being on mushrooms may induce these feelings that your brain can also attain naturally.

Our sense-of-self, or who we are, is predicated upon the identity we have crafted for ourselves. This is often based upon our experiences, life events, our personality and those around us. The way we see the world is through our own perspective; it is anchored in the 'ego' or the 'self'. Certain spiritualists are capable of dissolving their ego, and mushrooms can produce similar effects for some. Essentially, they can dissolve all we know to be real; our perception of reality and our sense or perception of self.

We now look at three different people's experiences of real people, and real experiences with nothing left out.

7

OBSERVING A TRIP: TRIP REPORTS

Sometimes the best wisdom comes from experience. But you don't need to experience it yourself to hear about it. We have summarised some trip reports from people who have documented their experiences through journaling. We have selected a few: those that are good, something in between and one that was a negative experiences.

We also took a pick of experiences that happened on varied doses, from 3.5 grams dried, to 10 grams fresh. Like people, every mushroom is different, and every trip varies from person-to-person. One running theme throughout is that mushrooms only work with what you already have. If you are in a bad place, a depressed or anxious state, they can lead to bad experiences, delusions, flashbacks or paranoia.

Someone who is generally well grounded and feeling positive will be more likely to have a more positive experience. If you are feeling rough or anxious, or convince yourself you won't have a good time, or go into the experience with anxiety, it is very likely that with mushrooms this will happen. If you think about it logically, mushrooms take you inward. If you feel ready to explore what's inside, the psychedelic experience could be an interesting one.

Mushrooms can create interesting visuals and distort reality in a physical, visual, way. Interestingly, none of our trip reports speak of visual alterations, rather, they emphasise the way people feel. Starting with a positive experience, this next section walks you through the ups and downs of tripping to give you some real insight.

Trip report one: A positive experience

This is about a spiritual journey from someone who is ready to face their inner-self and others with love.

From the 18th July 2018, an experienced mushroom taker (although he states it had been a while), took a dose of 3.5 grams and wrote about his experience from start to finish.

The author of "positive experience", workdoodler, had the house to himself after his wife and new baby had left for the weekend. The purpose of shrooms for him was a spiritual journey, and one of discovery. The intent of the drug taking seems to influence very much its outcome too.

As you will see throughout, this trip was largely positive, in contrast to the experience further on. Anxiety is common, so it is down to each person to know whether they are likely to be able to handle it or not. While he reports of a positive trip, like many trip journals, this one also reports of facing anxieties mid-way through. This journaler says he is sitting there, midtrip, "about to face MYSELF, MY ANXIETY". He has the mental elasticity to bring himself around though, oscillating back to "letting the negative go and the love overflow".

Trips often go in stages, with the mental state of the person tripping changing, and going in ebbs and flows. After the initial euphoria for this guy, the following part of the trip involved a large amount of introspective activity, internalizing, and caught up in thoughts. For some people, this is a positive and healthy experience. This guy stopped journaling for a time before coming back to his journal after an hour or so in his own thoughts, doing nothing. For the author of this trip report, mushrooms were spiritual and helped him realize a few things (at least at the time). He wrote:

"Through eating shrooms, I was looking for a 'spiritual journey', and I now realize that our lives ARE the spiritual journeys!". Breaking from ordinary thought patterns, mushrooms can have the effect of what is called "altering consciousness."

After various revelations about life and human nature, he went inward again, stopped journaling, and began doodling. Some revelations were more pertinent than others. He writes: "Always keep a RED pen on you! AND plenty of pens to share with fellow human beings". Unlike many other trip reports, this guy journals at the time, thus logging the different stages. Other reports were written retrospectively, but this is largely because they were relatively turbulent at the time.

Trip report two: riding the waves

This one is about the ups and downs of tripping through unexpected events.

This journaler too took 2.5 grams and experienced "unintended" consequences, making the point that, even if you are in a good place emotionally and mentally, things may occur while you are on magic mushrooms that can potentially induce some anxieties. His message is not to refrain from taking magic mushrooms, but to be prepared to "ride the waves", which is the title of his account on shroomery.org.

Unlike idealistic depictions in films or through popular culture, which can at times glamorize drugs, real experiences highlight the good and the bad, letting you make up your own mind. As journaler two shows, mushrooms confront the realities of the depths of your mind and the real world. After planning to trip and go straight to a dubstep gig, this journaler and his friend ended up downtown, tripping in a public place when their gig was canceled. Further still, in their "fragile states of mind" they ended up in a car collision. These guys kept their cool (just about) and concluded that:

"The trip could have gone seriously bad, in fact, it did for a short while, but as mush always does, it taught me something. From that point on I never take psychedelics for the visuals or the "high". I take them to ride out wherever it takes me and my unsuspecting mind. I don't fight the negative thoughts anymore, now I listen to them to see why they are there. Now explaining tripping to someone, visuals are the last thing I mention, not the first. Psychs can be so much more than what most people perceive them as. You just have to ride the waves and land ashore wherever they may take you."[8]

Trip report three: 'anxiety and mushrooms'

This journaler's trip triggered an anxiety attack and ongoing anxiety issues. It offers advice to see a psychologist or to know yourself before tripping.

This person published because they wanted to share their experience with people who have anxieties before taking psychedelics. They were nervous about having a bad trip but took "only ten grams fresh", they wrote. On the first trip, they had "insights and good thoughts for the last two hours", where they "spent most of it throwing a tennis ball at a wall and feeling good about it :)."

Their second trip led to a five-hour anxiety attack in wave after "wave of terror." This report highlighted some issues that resided with this person for five months afterwards: an anxiety disorder they had to seek psychiatric help for. While this person does not blame the mushrooms for the anxiety disorder, they do determine them as a trigger for it. This person, through their experience, offers the following advice:

"Personally, I would advise anyone before taking mushrooms to go visit a psychologist for a few sessions before and make sure you are not suffering from any pre-existing mental conditions. As an analogy, before supercharging your car make sure the engine is ok or it might blow up…"[9]

8
TRIP SITTING, TRIPPING SAFE AND MANAGING A BAD TRIP OR TRIPPER

We know mushrooms are illegal but it is worth knowing what to do, step-by-step if you have a bad trip or come across someone who is. Or maybe you have been picked to be a 'trip-sitter', a sound and measured sober friend who does not judge and keeps friends out of danger and in a happy, safe, space.

If you are having a bad trip:

1. Take deep breaths. Say: "it will pass, it will pass".

2. Close your eyes tightly and open them again.

3. Go and put some chill music on.

4. Have a nice cartoon cued up and ready to watch.

5. Distract yourself.

6. Get some fresh air (no where dangerous).

7. Take vitamin C or have a sugary drink.

. . .

If someone you know is having a bad trip, or you are trip sitting and someone reaches out:

1. Take them seriously but do not freak out. Listen and tell them to redirect their focus on something nice (it helps if you know the sort of things that are pleasant to experience whilst on mushrooms).

2. Put on some nice music (nothing too distorted, heavy or intense).

3. Don't give them any other drugs or anything. Do not encourage them to take more mushrooms.

4. Get some fresh air but stay safe.

5. If they are near an open window or anything else unsafe, remove them from danger and bring them back to safety, calmly telling them: "it will pass, time is moving on and this will all pass, I am here".

6. If they continue to behave in an unsafe way, or move towards traffic, or attempt to harm themselves and others, do not hesitate to call an ambulance or emergency services. Do not panic and know that mushrooms as a substance generally do not kill people and this is likely a panic attack that will pass.

9

WHAT DO THE RESEARCHERS SAY ABOUT THE EXPERIENCE?

The trip reports or case studies we looked at generally coincide with the academic literature. Research participants generally experienced the same cycles in changes of emotion, consciousness and perception over the course of four to six hours. Medium doses tend to lead to internalization or introspection, euphoria or dream-like states, synaesthesia and adjust perceptions of time and space.

Attention spans can be altered and the research states, like the trip reports above, there are oscillations from pleasant through to panic and dysphoric. Interestingly, the research also indicates that interpersonal support in a setting can reduce panic and increase positive experiences. In other words, tripping alone can be a dangerous business.

If you are going to take them, trip aware: know yourself and your surroundings. See our Do's and Don't section for safer tripping.

There has been some revised research into the controlled testing of the active properties of mushrooms and their potential benefits to jolt people out of addiction or mental health issues. The next section explores this. However, this next part should be read as rather separate to the recreational use of uncontrolled amounts of a drug in a domestic or social environment.

10

MUSHROOMS AND MENTAL HEALTH

The experiences of people on magic mushrooms, or tales of people 'going mad' after toxic doses, lead to a bit of a confusing picture. That is, if you throw the research about the potential benefits magic mushrooms have on mental health into the mix, you might see the two ideas as totally contradictory. Let's say, at this point, that there is a massive difference between drugs research in a controlled environment and buying something on the street from a person you don't know and taking them with friends.

Dr Philip Gerans, author of *The Measure of Madness: Philosophy of Mind, Cognitive Neuroscience, and Delusional Thought* (2014) and Chris Lethby who explores psychedelic drugs from a philosopher's point of view, recently teamed together to explore the way in which psychedelic drugs may have an impact on mental health disorders. [10]

This is the kind of research that can be extracted and misinterpreted as powerful sound bites that advocate the use of uncontrolled substances for mental health disorders. People should also be aware of the powerful warnings *against* using these drugs in an uncontrolled way to manage mental health disorders or anything similar. In fact, it is unwise to self-medicate, and experts actually warn against taking hallucinogens if you have a history of psychosis or other serious conditions, as our case studies above did demonstrate.

The following extract is about this study which simply looked at a controlled way that aspects of the drug's active properties may be used for positive gain. Headlines like this: "Active Ingredient in Shrooms Could 'Reset' Brains of Depressed People" from the subsection of Vice, certainly catch people's attention, but could be misleading without more context.

The basic premise in Geran's and Lethby's research is that psychedelic drugs like psilocybin mushrooms are transformative, and thus can provide a shock to the system, essentially rewiring the brain and assisting people with addiction or depression. While everyone experiences the world differently, we do so based upon patterns and models of the brain. The idea is that mushrooms can help to break these patterns of behavior and challenge the model to which we are bound. For example, if we are conditioned to be distrusting of others, the argument is psychedelic therapy could break these patterns.

A study from New York University also tested psilocybin-assisted therapy in a clinical trial. Researchers also interviewed thirteen adults who had previously taken part in a study.[11] Patients who reported anxiety at the start of the experience, all described a transformation in interpersonal relationships, and some felt a new connection with other humans and the rest of the world.

Seemingly, this is nothing new and has been experienced by many people taking mushrooms. The researchers of this study pointed out that very little had been done to explore the individual (subjective) experience of magic mushrooms and they believe that a combination of psilocybin along with psychotherapy could alleviate anxiety disorders.

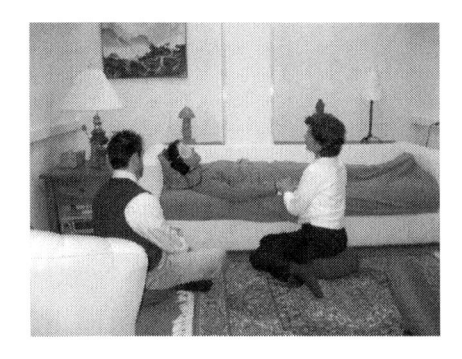

Figure 7. A psilocybin study session at John Hopkins. (Wikimedia)

However, for every argument for the potential benefits of this, there are many other counter-arguments. Generally speaking, as testified to in the trip reports you can find online, people with good mental health enjoy positive trips. Those with underlying anxieties should avoid psychedelic experiences altogether. And mushrooms and their doses of psilocybin, and the effects they have on mental health are unpredictable and uncontrolled. Researchers point out that testing drugs in a controlled way is not an endorsement for their recreational use but, maybe the Mexican healer Maria Sabina was onto something back in the 1950s.

11

FREQUENTLY ASKED QUESTIONS

These are all your frequently asked questions, at a glance.

Some of you might want a quick overview of mushrooms and tripping. While we in no way promote the use of illegal drugs, we all have a responsibility to know the facts.

Are mushrooms addictive?

No, mushrooms are generally not recorded as being addictive. Tolerance for mushrooms builds up after repeated usage so, generally speaking, mushrooms do not encourage repeated use in a short space of time. There is always the chance that you become addicted to the experience of tripping, taking mushrooms, or experimenting with them.

Some people develop a lifelong fascination with them, growing them or becoming experts on various strains, types and experiences. There are people who have made a career from this or have become expert bloggers, writers or scientists on the topic.

. . .

Are there drugs tests for magic mushrooms?

Psilocybin, the active properties in magic mushrooms, turns into psilocin. This can be found in urine and hair samples. Traces of magic mushrooms disappear pretty quickly. In urine, it is normally gone within a few hours, maximum 24 or, in cases of chronic doses or overuse, 48 hours. It can remain in your blood for 1-2 days but normally disappears pretty quickly compared to other substances.

How do magic mushrooms affect the brain?

Magic mushrooms affect the brain through the chemical compounds attaching themselves to serotonin (happy) receptors in the brain. They alter consciousness by disrupting thought patterns and changing the normal signal patterns around your brain, meaning that you perceive reality in a different way, often processing visual and sensory information in new ways.

Can magic mushrooms be spiked or laced?

Because of their appearance, they are unlikely to be cut with other drugs. However, some reports have suggested that normal mushrooms have been sold to unsuspecting people and that some of these are laced with LSD instead of organically containing the psychoactive properties of mushrooms, psilocybin. Also, if they are crushed and dried/in pill form, you will not know what is inside or whether they are cut with something else.

How long does a trip last?

A trip generally lasts between four to six hours when the mushrooms are eaten. It takes between thirty to sixty minutes to come up.

What do magic mushrooms look like?

With over 180 psilocybin containing mushroom species out there, it is impossible to summarise what magic mushrooms look like specifically. However, what they have in common is that they have a cap and a stem and gills underneath. Their color varies considerably. Many of them are very easily confused with poisonous varieties and spore prints have to be taken in order to identify them correctly.

How do magic mushrooms make you feel?

Magic mushrooms have an effect on the central nervous system. How they make you feel is very much dependent on you. They can induce euphoria-like feelings, visual sensations, an altered sense of time and space but also, in some cases, anxiety or nervousness.

Are magic mushrooms dangerous?

Magic mushrooms are generally considered 'safe' in chemical terms. Their danger lies in triggering psychotic episodes if you have mental health disorders. In very rare cases they can cause prolonged anxiety. They generally do not result in death unless dangerous activity is carried out whilst under the influence. They are not as known to cause flashbacks (as in the case of LSD).

How are mushrooms stored?

Once picked, mushrooms remain fresh from between five and ten days, depending entirely on their water content. You can store them in the fridge. However, like any living organism, they can rot if left longer. If not, you can put them into a container or sealed bag and freeze them for around seven months to one year. Many people choose to dry them for use much later on. This is most people's preferred option. Psilocybin mushroom potency is reduced through drying but not by a significant amount at all.

. . .

How do you dry mushrooms?

Drying them can be achieved by letting them air dry on a piece of paper or speeding up the process by drying them on a piece of paper on a radiator. After you have dried them, it is best to put them in an airtight container, although you should be aware that their strength will gradually decrease over time. You can also put them in an oven with the door open or in an oven with the door closed (as long as the temperature does not go over 95 Fahrenheit/ 36 degrees).

How do you prepare magic mushrooms?

This is entirely up to the person taking them but most people prefer tea as it is gentler on the stomach. Be careful not to boil the water but to just stew the mushrooms in warm water. You can add herbs, flavorings or herbal tea to improve on the taste. When mushrooms are picked fresh, they should be rinsed before consumption.

Can you eat mushrooms as they are?

Mushrooms are also eaten fresh or dried, however, this can cause stomach cramps and vomiting, and the taste is unpleasant, so most people prefer to brew tea.

How many magic mushrooms do you need to trip?

This is varied depending on the type/strain.

Liberty Caps dried require one to three grams for a medium dose, and three to seven for a strong dose, or two to eighteen fresh for a moderate trip and seven to forty two fresh for a strong one. *Cubensis* require one to three dried, or two to seven for a stronger trip. For *cubensis* that are fresh, the maximum dose for a very strong trip is up to twenty eight grams fresh. These are very rough guidelines.

. . .

What is it like to trip?

Tripping can be euphoric, visual and cause altered consciousness. Throughout the duration, you may oscillate between happy feelings, panicky, relaxed, insular, thoughtful and creative.

Should you take other drugs with mushrooms?

It is inadvisable to take other drugs with magic mushrooms. Some people take cannabis alongside it which they say can reduce sickness at the start for the first hour. However, cannabis can also increase anxiety and panic which could combine with the mushrooms. There are reports online of people going overboard and being pulled in many different directions by a cocktail of substances. Amphetamines (speed) and cocaine are especially to be avoided. They just don't go. We discuss this in more detail on the mixology section in this guide.

What do mushrooms do to the brain?

After the psilocybin is converted to psilocin in the body, it is pumped to the brain where it increases a type of serotonin (5HT-2A) – which controls the neural transmission of things affecting mood, perception, memory, awareness and appetite.

What are the after effects? (Comedowns)

After effects of mushrooms, comedowns, are not really a major feature of the drug. As we saw with trip report 3, some people experience psychological effects triggered by the mushrooms themselves, but there is nothing necessarily chemical that occurs. The day after taking mushrooms, people can generally feel tired or a little confused, or things and experiences that have occurred during the tripping itself can stay with you (good or bad). Comedowns as to the sort felt on ecstasy or MDMA are not as comparable.

12

BONUS CHAPTER: DO'S AND DON'TS

Here is our list of shrooming do's and don'ts. First and foremost make sure you know the legal guidelines of the country you're in ton taking magic mushrooms.

DO sort out your environment:

You are way more likely to have an enjoyable experience if you are in a good space.

1. Advice from seasoned trippers: clean the flat, house or room you are tripping in. You will find that dirtiness looks worse than ever, and even clean things will still look a little bit distorted and gross.
2. Make yourself a comfortable spot and keep things a nice temperature. The journey is supposed to be for your mind, you don't want to feel cold and edgy.

DON'T have any freaky posters around. If it freaks you out when you are sober, it will freak you out ten-fold if you take magic mushrooms

DO take a small dose to start with. Users say to take small amounts to see where you get on. Once they kick into your system, you can't remove them. We've gone through already how these organic drugs are an absolute lottery when it comes to dosage.

DO relax and go with it. Trip reporter number three tried to make herself sick to get rid of the effects but she had to ride out the trip for another four hours. Trip reporter number two said to be aware and ride the waves. Try your best to relax. Make sure you have the capacity to face your *known* anxieties and have the ability to calm yourself down *before* you even consider tripping, a bit like trip reporter number one.

DO listen to nice music. Queue up your playlist and avoid nasty surprises. Users have also noted that you might not even notice if the music has been off for a while!

DO enjoy the sun and fresh air in a safe environment.

DO get into a brilliant headspace before taking them. Mushrooms and bad trips can kind of work on a self-fulfilling prophecy basis.

DO write and journal to share your experiences.

DO NOT TAKE THEM IF:

. . .

You are naturally anxious and prone to panic attacks (or haven't had one before but think you could). Mushrooms are completely inadvisable. Why would you go somewhere that scares you? That is the trip you will have.

You or your family have a history of psychosis, paranoia or mental illness

Your friends convince you of it. This is a personal choice. Messing about with drugs is not cool when it goes completely wrong and you are left downtown with three people freaking out staring at their hands and unable to get into a cab.

You're in crappy company. If you are with someone who makes you feel uncomfortable, or edgy, or is generally a bit unsupportive, wait for another time altogether and do it with people who love you.

You are super young. You don't want to be messing with your brain while you are still growing and have a concoction of hormones going about. Just wait until you know yourself and feel comfortable in your own skin.

You are high already. Panic and paranoia strike fast…why mess with that mix?

Other Tips

DO stay informed. Read, read, read! There are tons of trip reports online. Avoid the fake and glamorized blogs, and go for the real, raw, unedited, versions

. . .

DO make good decisions about where to trip before you start. If you start off indoors, you are likely to stay safe. While there are no real incidents of deaths *because* of the substance in mushrooms, there are tons of reports out there about excessive and toxic doses (hard to regulate) leading to death, criminal activity and all sorts of horrors.

DON'T go picking random mushrooms. You **don't know** what you're doing, and a small change in gill spacing, stem size or an invisible change in spore print, can result in death.

DON'T break the law. You can go on mushroom retreats to countries where the law is more relaxed.

DO look after your fellow trippers.

DO get a trip sitter, a sober person who will look after you.

DO love yourself and others, no matter what.

AFTERWORD

Hopefully, you have enjoyed this explorer's guide, and it has met your curiosity for information on magic mushrooms.

We definitely journeyed through time and explored the human relationship with magic mushrooms. We saw trip reports from 9000 years ago on a cave wall and the first viral trip report that sparked the whole hippie movement towards hallucinogens.

We took a tour of mushroom prep, dangers, and benefits of magic mushrooms according to some pretty radical research in the making.

We shared three diverse experiences and invite you to share and read more. Attached are resources if you'd like to do some further readings and want to discover more about this fascinating drug.

ALSO BY ALEX GIBBONS

Did you enjoy the book or learn something new? It really helps out small publishers like Alex if you could leave a quick review on Amazon so others in the community can also find the book!

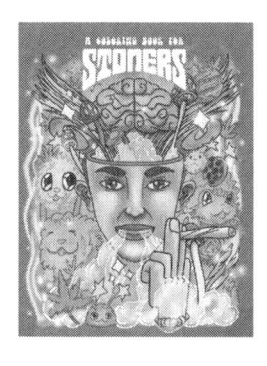

★★★★★

―――

Want to chill and experience the benefits of mindfulness? Want to do something productive while watching random videos on YouTube?

Get this fun stoner themed coloring book to scribble on for your next trip. Search for 'Alex Gibbons Stoner Coloring Book' on Amazon to get yours now!

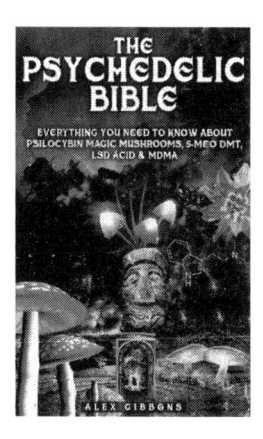

―――

Thinking about taking other magical drugs? Ever wondered what exactly happens when you take them? Want to make sure you don't have a bad trip?

If you want to read more about the history, origins and effects of Magic Mushrooms, LSD/Acid or DMT, search for 'The Psychedelic Bible' on Amazon!

For daily posts on all things Psychedelic, follow us on Instagram @Psychedelic.curiosity

PART II

ACID THE TRUTH ABOUT LSD

A STAY SAFE GUIDE TO LYSERGIC ACID DIETHYLAMIDE

Taking LSD was a profound experience, one of the most important things in my life.

— Steve Jobs

13
WHAT IS LSD?

LSD - mind-altering civilization

LSD is the prime substance that ignited the modern wave of interest towards psychedelics and the revolution of consciousness of worldwide proportions. The impact of lysergic acid on the human culture is unprecedented, as it not only boosted a mass appeal towards mind-altering compounds, but it also brought in mainstream forgotten aboriginal cultures and their knowledge of medicinal rituals with trance plants.

Therefore, we could say that LSD turned the page, expanding people's drive for enlightenment practices, as well as for a completely different approach to reality. With the experience of LSD, the practical industrialized society was beginning to search for meaning in the fantastic and symbolic realms.

The times synchronized perfectly such as to confer the optimal context for the LSD wave to emerge. In a social atmosphere affected by the recently passed World Wars, with the industrial revolution on the rise and the other smaller yet tormenting wars, like the Vietnam War, maintaining a status quo of general conflict and pressure, a shock that would shatter the conventional and bring new intelligence in the game was most welcomed.

The hippie movement offered fertile grounds for the culture of psychedelics to grow into a veritable culture. Peace and enlightenment were sought for in Eastern spirituality, as well as in the instant effect of psychedelic drugs and further on in South America's rituals of healing and spirit connection.

Lysergic acid funnels the bonding with nature but, at the same time, is a synthetic compound and thus could be seen as the link between the contemporary mechanized society and Mother Earth. As other psychedelics, it amplifies the senses and expands the area of perception in that you see more, hear more, and feel intense detail. This is partly the source of fascination towards the world and life overall that one remains with as an aftereffect of LSD.

The sensation is that you are perceiving the divine and, at the same time, being conscious of its presence within. This is a truly revolutionary mindset in the context of the traditionalist society that survived a world crisis and was brought, with the aid of psychedelics, in the middle of the modern renaissance.

It was LSD that sparked the appetite for the unknown realities of the hallucinogenic states, because acid was something very different. It induced a sort of lightness of being instead of the, more often than not, heavy trip of the magic mushrooms or the other psychotropic plants that usually provoked a trance.

Furthermore, LSD had a more digital effect. It didn't present the usual hallucinations of mythical animals, fairies, monsters, or whatever creatures dwelled in the collective imaginarium. Its effect was to reveal the image of vibrations, the vibration of sound and light that received form, as well as objects that were seemingly inanimate, like rocks or furniture.

It was thus opening the eyes to the life that inherently is in everything, infusing the reality that we all perceive in a similar way with spirit. For all these reasons, LSD was the perfect substance to attract and awaken the enthusiasm.

The consumerist trend, in part, diluted the initial revelations, as with the advance in the discovery and research of psychotropic substances, a great number of psychedelic acids emerged and were brought into the market. Different types of acids soon became recreational party drugs, the next generation changing the purpose of use, as well as the essential meaning behind the experience this substance induced.

Nonetheless, the tribal gatherings of today are marked by the feeling of communion between people and a profound connection with nature, the blueprints of the original psychedelic experience and the powerful collective insights that were the gift of LSD.

In addition, lysergic acid is in the midst of a new revival, since the recent medical studies have exposed its therapeutic potential and accustomed its use to the system of efficiency and alert rhythm characterizing our current society by introducing microdosing. This method of consuming LSD became popular in a short while, being the optimal solution for busy people.

An artificial compound coming from a natural source

Despite the fact that LSD's most usual presentation is on small paper stamps that have been soaked in the substance, its source is natural. Lysergic acid is extracted from a fungus that develops on rye seeds. In other words, it's the rot of a type of cereal that produces this mind-bending effect on human consciousness. Of course, one cannot consume the rotten rye and expect to have anything else but poisoning.

In support of this idea, there are several incidents that have been registered in the course of history, one of which is famous: the intoxication of an entire village in the 50's in France with the addled flour that the sole baker of the place had used to make bread for the population. The event is chronicled, but the circumstances in which such a large mass of people were poisoned are still unelucidated, especially as the effects were horrific and ended up with loss of human lives. Nonetheless, this type of event has added another dimension to the mythical image of the substance, more so as the intoxicated men presented the effects of strong hallucinations.

From another point of view, LSD presents yet another set of peculiarities: it is taken in very small doses of 100-400 micrograms, which means the extraction has to be highly diluted. It can penetrate the skin barrier and enter the bloodstream directly, lasting anywhere from 4-6 hours, where the experience is so powerful that its aftereffects can be sensed weeks, months, and even a year later.

When talking about LSD's effect of opening a gate towards interconnectivity with nature, with everything and everybody, with the universe, we should mention that this is, in fact, the action that this substance has on the neurons of the brain. It is like turning on the light in the neural network, freeing and activating all circuits. An enhancement in perception and a leap of consciousness are only natural results of these processes.

For this reason, the notion that LSD alters the mind doesn't seem to grasp fully its encompassing influence, for the state of awareness is not bent but rather more comprehensive, present, and dynamic. Its effect is one of resetting the pre-existent predicament in which the brain functions, giving a restart to all connections and inducing a full-power operating mode.

Subsequently, it's for these incredible abilities that lysergic acid is studied as a therapeutic solution for a number of mental conditions, such as addiction, depression, anxiety, and post traumatic stress disorder (PTSD).

14

THE HISTORY AND CULTURAL INFLUENCE OF LSD

Prior to LSD's synthesization, there have been documented cases of poisoning with rye and wheat that have gone bad. Lysergic acid is naturally occurring in ergot, a by-product of the infection with a fungus that turns the kernels of the cereals black. One of its horrific effects, if eaten, results in the rotting of the person's limbs and their subsequent coloring, turning them black.

In one circumstance around 1700, a family was poisoned and died, whereas around the mid-twentieth century in France, a whole village was intoxicated; several people died while others remained marked for life with severe physical and mental conditions. In all cases, apart from the rapid decay of the flesh, there were other symptoms that resemble much more what we know about LSD today, vivid hallucinations and delusions.

Given the combined effect that the ergot fungus had on the human body, as well as the abnormal, unassumed context in which this happened, the behavior of those inflicted was rather strange and violent. To add to this myth, there is a theory that states the famous Salem witch trials were a consequence of such poisoning of the population, during a highly rainy, wet summer that favoured the development of the fungus on the cereal used as food.

Although we are more or less discussing the same chemical compound, our firm knowledge of lysergic acid begins with the Swiss chemist Albert Hoffman on his bicycle ride home. It spans over a very short period compared to other psychedelics that have been used for millennia, defining the modern era of substances.

Short historic timeline of LSD

Albert Hoffman was researching a substance that would aid pregnant women with uterine contractions during childbirth. He synthesized the compounds from the ergot, obtaining a long list of lysergic acid derivatives, of which LSD was the 25th, hence its original naming as LSD-25.

This happened in 1938, but as he didn't find anything that seemed to be useful for his purpose, he put all the research in a drawer and left it on standby. It wasn't until 1943, when he thought he'd give it another shot, that he sent the substance to the pharmacological department for analysis.

Before doing this, Hoffman resumed the process of synthesizing, and the magical error occurred when a very small drop accidently fell on his skin. He went on without noticing the incident, but at a certain point during the work, he noticed that he was 'affected by a remarkable restlessness, combined with a slight dizziness' that compelled him to take the day off and go home (as he confesses in his book 'LSD, My Problem Child').

The aforementioned famous bicycle ride follows, and then, once in the intimacy of his house, he calmly gives off to the pleasant sensation of intoxication that was inducing a dreamlike state in which his imagination ran vividly, producing the now all-familiar visual patterns of kaleidoscopic pictures, mandalas, and distortions of vibration. This was the first trip on LSD that a human being had experienced, and it lasted about two hours.

The experience sparked his interest, so he submitted the compound to his laboratory at Sandoz to inquire further, carrying out tests on animals that would define its toxicity, tolerance, and other properties. The research continued with studies of its effects on human beings in a psychiatric environment, on schizophrenic and healthy individuals that, even though came out with no specific result in terms of therapeutic benefits, still remained a substantial promise.

The similarity of its effects with certain types of psychosis was the point of attraction for the psychiatrists that experimented further to establish its influence, but no evident correlation was determined. Nonetheless, during the '50s and '60s, LSD was the prime drug used in hallucinogenic assisted therapy. A great volume of documentation was produced in the medical research of lysergic acid, and over 40,000 people were prescribed this substance for therapeutic purposes.

The amazing effect that LSD had on the human brain generated a wave of enthusiasm among a different group of people, particularly among the brilliant minds of the day that were rather interested in its influence on consciousness. Starting with the psychologist Timothy Leary, who eventually became the star of the psychedelic revolution, a series of cultural personalities were invited to take part in assisted LSD experiments and afterwards to share and spread the insights they were granted.

These were the first steps that were taken by the elite of the pre-hippie period and the most important basis for the new consciousness revival that was to take up the whole world. Leary was prophesying 'Turn on, tune in, and drop out', words that would become a meme of the counterculture rising in those moments in the USA and spreading across the globe as a response to the pre-established blueprint of reality that was getting too tight and abusive for a generation of enlightened spirits.

At the same time, the secret services around the world were indulging in all sorts of mind control experiments, using with predilection amphetamines and mescaline. In this type of pursuit, the CIA started its research LSD as part of the controversial work performed by the Project MKULTRA, inquiring on its capacity to become some sort of truth serum.

Under the umbrella of top-secret operations, lysergic acid was administered to hundreds of men, including military employees and agents, as well as individuals from the general public, especially from the disadvantaged layers of society, like homeless people, prostitutes or delinquents, of which most were given the substance without knowledge or consent. It was a wild type of research that evidently produced no solid results apart from the terrorizing of those individuals, and the project officially ended in the mid 1970s.

Under these predicaments and inflated by the overall hype of the hippie movement, the use of LSD peaked in the 60s and 70s, transforming into a veritable hysteria. A veil of unconsciousness dominated the consumption of LSD during that period, and although there was a powerful trend involving awareness and enlightenment, there were numerous cases of people taking lysergic acid in contexts and settings that were definitely unfavorable, ending in nervous collapses, violent accidents, criminality, and suicide. All of these events were, of course, exploited by the media, damaging the public image of LSD and instating this substance as a dangerous drug.

Consequently, in 1970, LSD was declared a Schedule I drug with high potential for abuse and wasn't accepted for further research into its therapeutic benefits. This decision would halt the study of lysergic acid for many years in the USA, as well as in other parts of the world.

As of the 1980s, however, the interest reemerged in the recreational usage of LSD, as well as in the science of its therapeutic properties, and studies on its beneficial influence were resumed by newly formed organizations, such as MAPS (the Multidisciplinary Association of Psychedelic Studies) and The Beckley Foundation.

LSD is still popular among young people who consume it for amusement, but more so within ceremonial tribal gatherings that define the current new-age movement and individuals engaged in a personal pursuit of therapy or consciousness discovery. As for the medical scene nowadays, the interest in LSD is concentrated on its use in micro doses to support therapy.

The cultural revolution and Mckenna's take on LSD

All public figures that raised the idea to promote the spectacular effects that psychedelics had on the dynamics of the human brain were constantly persecuted; Timothy Leary, the father of the LSD movement, spent many years of his life in jail. The whole psychedelic culture ended up discredited by the media and oppressed by laws. Nonetheless, its aficionados were not only the hippies or, later on, the ravers, but an entire palette of individuals that one would surely not consider drug abusers.

They were scientists, business men, artists, people working in IT, politicians, doctors, and the list could go on indefinitely, citing people that led normal lives and actively participated in society. The enlightenment was there for anybody who had the courage and curiosity to delve into it. Moreover, in time, as the '60's revolutionary spirit mellowed, the psychedelics received a different glow, a more science-infused image that shed the conflict with establishment issues and established their presentation as guides to the subtle realms of reality and towards self-discovery and self-therapy.

Terence Mckenna inherited the legacy of Timothy Leary and further promoted the culture of psychedelics into the new era. He had entered the movement with a wild and essential step, praising the influence of magic mushrooms in our culture. In fact, the widespread consumption of psychedelic mushrooms is almost in its whole attributed to Terence and Dennis Mckenna, who developed a method to grow Stropharia cubensis, a type of mushroom that he became acquainted with in Colombia and introduced in mass to USA.

But more than developing a practical guide that supported the in-house growing of the mushrooms, he came up with a theory that stated they were, in fact, magical entities that had an essential role in the development of human culture over millennia and the evolution of our species. He was thus portraying psychedelics as a primordial element for human growth, one that was there with us all along and that was necessary and only natural to inquire further.

In Mckenna's opinion, going through life without psychedelics would resemble a life without sex. This was because the psychedelic compounds were the source of knowledge, of the laws that govern reality and the cosmos, the main source of novelty throughout our history, through the different types of plants people practiced with in all cultures of the globe. His approach was merging the tribal consciousness and know-how with the modern technologies and visions of the future.

With a degree in shamanism and ecology, Mckenna believed that bridging the old and new worlds was the key to a complete vision of humanity in which the missing evolutionary link that everybody was searching for was to be found in psychedelics. The door to understanding the ancient past civilizations, the meaning of life and means to make a sense out of the universe lay in entheogens.

Most fascinatingly, the psychedelic substances were leading to an enhanced system of perception in which the purest religious experience was the same thing as the encounter with pagan mythological characters and, at the same time, with the most bewildering science fiction scenarios.

What led him to the intense and exhaustive study of psychedelic substances and experiences was not the recreational use of drugs but the interest in the variety of religious experiences and different ways in which to grasp the understanding of human consciousness.

Aldous Huxley's book 'The doors of Perception' was, for Mckenna, the introduction into the wild world of the collective imaginarium, and from that moment, he started to develop his theory of the necessity and imminence of an archaic revival, a rebirth of the lost knowledge of human civilizations, those that went extinct along with the tribal counterpart that, although in a symbolic manner, kept the information well-hidden in their traditions. He believed these essential insights could and should be accessed through psychedelic experiences.

The first time Mckenna took acid was in 1965, a batch produced by Sandoz, in a dose of 500 micrograms, which is a serious quantity, rapidly expelling all preconceived ideas that one retains in terms of what's real and what's not. His words on this initial experience: 'It was a whole universe that polarized itself into two concepts. One was like God - it was profound. It was that organ tone in the Bach B minor Mass (...) then the other thing was hilarious and absurd and it caused me to bust up hysterically for long minutes. I spent an hour and a half in this place just ricocheting between things so awesome that I felt like a flea in God's bedroom.'

But Mckenna confesses that he appreciates LSD in its whole potential only when he combines it with hashish because, by itself, lysergic acid is not the type of substance to produce mind-blowing visions with flying dragons or his beloved 'elf machines' that dwelled in the high realms mastered by DMT.

LSD is only enhancing the perception of reality and, of course, leaving your imagination free to encounter whatever beings from outer space you'd wish to meet, but it does not force the introduction of such mystical guides. It's only you in the LSD trip; your consciousness is your sole guide, contrary to psilocybin, ayahuasca, or other plant entheogens that are always accompanied with a specific guide to take you on an insightful journey. In other words, Mckenna was in the search of mythological and science-fiction fairy tales, and the only way he could satisfy his need with LSD was to combine it with generous doses of hashish.

For Mckenna, the exploration of psychedelics is a way to prepare yourself for death, a means through which you go past the limits of the event horizon into the great unknown through the deepest meditation process one is able to induce while still alive.

Terence Mckenna was one of the world's greatest visionaries, the one who introduced the term 'psychonaut' to define the explorers of consciousness and recuperate this holy pursuit from the shame of the public opinion that denigrated its purpose, considering it mere addiction.

He died of a brain tumour that, despite the rumors, could've been the effects of a life-long consumption of drugs, but as doctors told him, was only nature and its intricate ways of messing with people lives. He spent his last days answering the thousands of fan emails and contemplating the mysteries of life and death, something he did during his entire existence.

15

THE SCIENCE BEHIND LSD

Chemistry of LSD

LSD is, in chemical terms, lysergic acid diethylamide, part of the great family of indole alkylamines, including tryptamines, such as psilocin, the active substance in magic mushrooms, or N,N-dimethyltryptamine or DMT. LSD is found on blotters, stamp-like pieces of paper submerged in acid, microdots, or small tablets and dissolved in solutions of water or alcohol.

Lysergic acid is synthesized from the ergot, the fungus of the rye, called C. purpurea, and its chemical appearance is that of a tetra-cyclic ring ($C_{20}H_{25}ON_3$). A number of homologs and derivatives have been studied, but none has been found to be as potent as LSD. One of its most familiar siblings is LSA, the substance extracted from the seeds of the Morning Glory.

The regular dosage is between 100 and 400 micrograms. A dose of 25 micrograms is expected to ignite visible effects when consumed, but the moderate dosage that would allow the full spectrum of potential is 75-150 micrograms. It alters perception by infusing the person with a state of euphoria and promoting one's inner capacity for introspection and for discerning the hypnagogic coordinates and dreams.

One may experience pseudo-hallucinations, so-called because they are not visions of non-existing characters and events but enhancements of perception of external stimuli that are there in reality. Synesthesia and the distortion of the time and space dimension describes what people may be tempted to define as illusion.

Pharmacology of LSD

One hypothesis that explains the effects of LSD on the human consciousness is that the brain experiences an informational overload of the senses. The usual functioning mode of our mind to select the needed sensory information and thus avoid overload of unnecessary stimuli and redundant information simply does not have a path to be transferred from reception to cognition.

The apparatus that performs the selection of perceived information is the thalamus, a ball of neurons in the center of our brain that decides what is relevant for us to know and what should be neglected from our exterior environment. LSD enables the thalamus to do its job properly; thus, a great wave of information penetrates the mind, pushing the brain into an overwhelming state in which it has to deal with greater input coming from its senses. This state of overload is what we decipher as a psychedelic state of mind.

Moreover, LSD has been found to interfere with the production of serotonin, and it's believed this neurotransmitter is also influencing the thalamus, interfering with the function of selecting the proper information from the outside medium. To study if serotonin is a key factor of the cortex overload, Katrin H. Peller from the University Hospital for Psychiatry Zurich experimented with a substance that would block the serotonin receptors.

The research was done on subjects that were administered LSD and ketanserin, the respective blocker. The results were surprising, as the people who were given this duo did not present the usual psychedelic effects of the acid. Further, the conclusions of the experiment stated that, by impeding the thalamus from performing the process of selection, awareness is shifted to a specific part of the brain, which is the posterior cingulate cortex.

Other studies revealed that LSD resets the pre-existing neural connections by creating new branches between neighboring cells, or in other words, greatly enlarging the number of pathways the brain uses when perceiving and disseminating the exterior information, as well as its capacity to reorganize the information that's already in the memory.

16

THE EFFECTS OF LSD

The LSD trip lasts 6-12 hours, depending on the dosage and the intensity of the journey. The live memory of the state lingers for weeks after, while the after-effect of a powerful LSD experience can be sensed throughout the rest of your lifetime.

The overstimulation of the senses that results in a general overload of the brain alters the normal perception of reality, enhancing emotions and producing an overwhelming avalanche of thoughts. This is the cause of the impression of hallucinating, where you think you see things that are not there when you're merely getting far more impressions from the existing reality. With this ultra-sensibilization, the information coming from the senses is often misinterpreted, and in some cases, the senses become confused, producing a state of synesthesia, where sounds produce forms and forms have different tastes.

The world appears in much more vivid colors, vibrations become visible, shapes get distorted, sometimes morphing one from another, and halos of light give the impression that you can discern the auras of things and beings. Hearing is also highly augmented; therefore, people consuming LSD testify to hearing sounds with more acuity, from a long distance and with a definition that allows great many details to penetrate the perception barrier.

Although one may experience a rapid shift in moods, the general state is one of euphoria, with dream-like experiences in an atmosphere of overall awareness and peacefulness. When the brain is totally overwhelmed, it's natural sometimes to become stuck in old mental patterns and refuse the experience, in which case the whole trip takes a turn towards confusion and ultimately anxiety. This scenario is the one of a classical bad trip that you can only avoid by freeing your mind of the usual expectations.

By inducing this altered sense of perception, lysergic acid messes with one's capacity to recognize and understand reality. One of the most often met consequences is a detachment from the self, by separation from your old belief system. This is what defines a transcendental experience in which time appears as a continuum, cold and hot are regarded as mere states of being, the borders between what seems to be a dream and what was, until that moment, stable reality, dissolves.

The feeling is of profound merging with everything that is within, comprising yourself and everything that lies outside, constituting the external environment. The dissolution of the self turns into a sense of community with oneself, as well as with everything there is. Peace, forgiveness, compassion, and an overwhelming sensation of unconditional love are the feelings a person on LSD experiences and the ultimate definition of a spiritual awakening.

Interfering with the levels of serotonin in the body, LSD is directly influencing the perception and behavior of the person, as well as the regulatory systems, such as hunger, temperature, motor control, and sexuality. But it goes even further by having a powerful impact on the emotional dimension of the individual: one can feel several emotions at the same time and swing rapidly from one emotional state to another. The confusion of senses, perception, and the emotional overrun could be disconcerting for some.

The effects of LSD linger on when the trip is finished, maintaining its memory through the recurrence of flashbacks. The after-effects are the increase of confidence, appetite for life, and focus on what is truly meaningful for one's being, thus generating important decisions and concrete changes in the long term. LSD also eliminates or considerably reduces addiction by revealing that we don't really need such attachments to clarify one's purpose in life.

We can also talk about the effects of a bad trip that erupt, as mentioned above, when one refuses to shift its pre-existing standpoint and actually accept the trip that LSD proposes. In these cases, panic, paranoia, and psychosis are waiting in line. As an after-effect, it can degenerate into a state of strong fatigue, aching body and muscles, insomnia, and depression, but this is only the consequence of not being able or open enough to assume the greatness of reality and existence.

These are also the fallouts of treating this powerful psychedelic substance with disrespect and mixing it with other drugs like amphetamines or alcohol. Also, not paying attention to the most important principle of 'set and setting' can severely disrupt your journey. The ambiance of a club or an environment of noise, agitation, crowds, unfamiliar grounds, and unfamiliar people, a context that is provoking anxiety are not the proper settings for a peaceful and insightful LSD trip. In the same line of thought, the interior setting is as important, whereas a state of mind of confusion, depression, or nervousness is not a fertile medium for enlightenment or a firm basis for self-discovery.

A regular intake of LSD creates tolerance that makes users increase the dosage; however, a break of a short period generally solves the problem. A typical LSD trip is so powerful that one generally needs a few months to integrate the insights and implement the beneficial understandings in their daily routine and in the dynamic of their life before they choose to take it again.

17
THE THERAPEUTIC POTENTIAL OF LSD

Due to LSD's capacity to induce special states of mind in which the person is faced with a powerful feeling of interconnection, as well as profound spiritual experiences, this substance is seen as a reliable solution for helping people that deal with life-threatening illnesses or conditions and that suffer from anxiety. The after-effects of using LSD support these purposes by promoting one's self-confidence, personal growth, belief systems, and confidence.

The manner in which LSD, as well as other psychedelics, work is by restructuring the brain, addressing particularly the dysfunctional mental patterns and the ideas and emotions that aren't in congruence with the rest of your being. The feeling of interconnectivity and union, as reflected within, is the catalyzer of containing the whole of yourself and thus accepting yourself for who you are, addressing your problems with courage, honesty and compassion, and maintaining an attitude of clarity and peace. LSD is promoting an uplifting perspective on life and a healthy approach of the individual path, which sustains the process of cleansing and renewal. In this course, issues and features that are unnecessary are eliminated; the burdens transform into practical tasks that, once resolved, give way to ease and freedom.

The feeling of communion is also associated with the sensation of detachment from the ego. One feels united with every atom of the universe and, by this, is freed from the attachment to his rigid system of beliefs, as well as to his specific problems. This is a natural consequence of being compelled to see the definition of the cosmos, the grand picture in all its complexity, instead on focusing exclusively on your own universe. You could say you have the opportunity to experience your smallness in the greatness of the universe.

The current research and experimental trials that are conducted to determine LSD's therapeutic abilities are based on the preliminary studies from the 1950-1960 period, when lysergic acid was considered helpful in the treatment of addiction, PTSD, depression, and anxiety. The procedure is to administer LSD to the patient while the therapist takes the role of the shaman, who guides and confers a feeling of comfort and security, while addressing the cause of his problems, the motif that ultimately sent him to therapy in the first place.

Under LSD, the patient is in an altered state of consciousness in which he can easily access his true self and work on his persona if the right instruments are found or handed to him. The experience has the form of a dream or trance that is greatly infused with symbolism and the figures of the unconscious, but at the end, the work that's been done has tremendous effects. Despite the way we forget dreams and despite the experience of other psychoactive substances, such as DMT, you will probably remember every detail of the LSD trip, a feature that enhances the benefits of such a journey.

Today, therapists, self-proclaimed, non-conventional, or with traditional degrees, are pursuing therapy with LSD, giving lysergic acid to their patients to treat their medical conditions or aid their personal development pursuit. Although not legal, these people play the roles of the modern urban shamans, performing their work with perseverance and a great dose of awareness, promoting their practice by word of mouth from one satisfied patient to the other.

Most of them have normal jobs and live a normal life, and there's no evident reason to suspect something from their appearance or their overall behavior. The current laws, however, would punish such actions severely, as LSD is considered dangerous for abuse, so giving LSD to others would almost be an act of violence. Moreover, the social predicament is as unfriendly with such therapies, for the media took care to portraitize acid as a cause of numerous accidents, delinquency and crimes, as part of the denigration campaign of the 'war on drugs'. Nonetheless, there are more and more people that take part in such private sessions with lysergic acid, people that are suffering from different conditions or in pursuit of discovery and spirituality as seen from a non-conventional point of view.

Studies

To this day, the research and experimental trials that have been done concerning the use of LSD as medicine for a number of mental conditions are still too few and, in some aspects, inconclusive enough to funnel the therapeutic implementation on a mass scale. Most materials were produced during the 50s, 60s, 70s, and it's only recently that the active interest of conventional medicine towards lysergic acid has reemerged.

The long period of pause due to the legal restraints made it even harder to regroup and restart the clinical investigations of LSD. Nonetheless, there is sufficient evidence to bring LSD into therapy again, more so in the cases where the pressure of time makes the difference, such as terminal stages of illnesses, because the beneficial effects of the therapy with LSD are manifesting immediately, but existing therapeutical means need a lot longer to produce relevant transformations in the patient's life.

A study conducted in London by R. Carhart-Harris, M. Kaelen, M. Bolstridge, T. Williams, L. Williams, R. Underwood, D. Nutt, titled 'The paradoxical psychological effects of lysergic acid diethylamide (LSD)' (2016) concluded that LSD could offer a promising treatment for depression and anxiety. The experimentation was performed on healthy individuals that were given a single dose of

LSD, and the results showed the experience provided them with an after-effect of optimism, openness, and an uplifted mood for up to two weeks after the session.

A similar study by T. Krebs and P-O Johansen, termed 'LSD for alcoholism' (2012), addressed the problem of alcohol addiction and the beneficial results. People that participated in this trial exhibited the same feeling of optimism and a boost of confidence that conferred the necessary power to face their alcohol problem and deal with it on a psychological, as well as practical, level.

Furthering Mckenna's view of LSD as a means to get acquainted with death, ultimately challenge and make peace with this primordial fear, research has been done in the quest of alleviating the anxiety of people that were dealing with terminal diseases. Among the studies performed in this sector, there is one very compelling trial conducted by P. Gasser, K. Kirchner, T. Passie, 'LSD-assisted psychotherapy for anxiety associated with a life-threatening disease: A qualitative study of acute and sustained subjective effects' (2015). It visibly reduced the level of anxiety produced by the fear of dying, not only by introducing them to the unknown, but also by supporting relaxation and improving their strength and ability to cope with the ending of life as they know it. The inquiry registered the after-effects lasting for a period of about a year.

There are also reports from celebrities that participated in LSD therapy, such as Cary Grant, the famous movie star, who was one of the first to be treated with lysergic acid. He did the therapy in 1958, taking one hundred doses over a period of three years. His testimony is that LSD helped him resolve childhood traumas and difficult relationship issues that he'd been carrying around for a lifetime. Acid brought him peace, the power of acceptance, and clarity of vision.

Microdosing

The hype of the moment is microdosing psychedelics, and LSD is preeminently leading the way. This method of using acid fits perfectly with today's society that lives in a highly alert rhythm and is in the search of remedies that would not impede their activity or produce a shock that could slow them down, make them lose focus, and make them less efficient. The interesting fact is that, in microdoses, LSD is helpful especially in those aspects, bringing on clarity and productivity.

Microdosing is done with 10 micrograms every fourth day, as prescribed by its pioneer James Fadiman. The usual effects of LSD are not apparent when using this method as the dose is too small to produce any type of sensible sensation. But its after-effects, on the other hand, can be sensed starting with day two and are manifested through a set of positive changes in behavior and state of mind, including the power of concentration, an uplifted mood, a boost in energy that generates productive activity, clarity and balance, and enhanced sense of confidence.

The medical research on microdosing is extremely scarce, but the internet is abundant with stories from people that have pursued this type of treatment, and their testimonies are extremely positive. Moreover, the microdosing craze has just begun.

18

PROS AND CONS OF LSD

As you've seen by now, there's a variety of ways in which a person can consume LSD. Therefore, the benefits and negative aspects depend on the purpose with which you take the drug. It is evident that it depends greatly whether you use LSD therapeutically, in a process of healing or growing yourself, or just to have fun one night at a party.

As a general rule, psychedelics are substances that generate an introspective process in which you travel within, so they are to be taken in environments that offer the necessary intimacy to be free to go along with the trip. When you get interrupted by the exterior realm or are in the pressure of maintaining your focus outside yourself, it is most likely that you will get stressed and respond negatively to that stimuli.

The state of being when on LSD is susceptible to changes and getting disrupted is reflected in the overall harmony of the trip. You are also highly empathic and feeling all vibrations from outside manifesting strongly inside yourself. For this reason, the environments with big crowds and agitated spirits would most likely provoke tension within you; taking a trip and going for a walk on a busy street would be like going to the circus for the first time.

We discussed earlier the problem of set and setting, outlining that it is highly important to choose the proper ambience and enter a state of mind in which you are prepared for the journey, because it actually makes the difference between a good and a bad trip. LSD is an incredibly relative drug, so when facing anxiety or panic attacks, being under pressure for whatever reason, tired or troubled, nervous or agitated, it would be wise to postpone the trip because its effect would be immensely influenced.

Furthermore, it comes down to compatibility. The experience of LSD is inevitably astounding for everybody that tries it, but for some, it is so pleasurable and useful that they engage in a regular therapy or self-therapy, while for others, it's too disruptive to do it again. As such, it is a matter of your psychological and emotional structure, of acceptance and flexibility.

So, apart from the potential of a bad trip, there is no real con. But this doesn't mean you have to underestimate a bad trip as its aftereffects can be devastating and long term. Mental conditions and past traumas can be healed with LSD therapy, but they can also be aggravated when the consumption is unconscious, unguided, or unprepared. A weak, unsure, and troubled person can be seriously affected, and the inability to face and control the manifestation of the effects and aftereffects of the trip can be tormenting, rooting the individual even more into their problems.

On the other hand, it is only when we truly face our fears and suffering that we become free and are able to reach above the surface of our issues, and LSD is evidently a great support in this direction. But for such beneficial, life-changing results, you need courage, perseverance, or the proper guide who knows what they're doing.

One of the biggest risks of taking LSD today is when buying it on the street and not from a reliable source that can attest to its purity. There's a high chance you'd not be given lysergic acid but another strain. There are a plethora of derivatives and other types of substances and psychedelic compounds that, from a chemical point of view, are considered acids but not LSD exactly. LSD is the most famous and the purest of them all, and due to this, there are many occasions when other types of substances are sold under its name.

The reasons are multiple, yet it's most likely that they're easier to produce and use cheaper ingredients and equipment. Most frequent acids that are passed on as LSD are Shulgin's recipes 2CI, 2CE, and 2CB. Even though they're definitely rougher, they do have an enlightening aspect if you manage to get through the first stages of pure madness and surrender your attachments to any fixed structures of perception.

Unfortunately, there is a list of other acids that you would never want to try, and you can stumble upon them anywhere, hidden in the same presentation as LSD, minuscule stamps with beautiful colorful prints on them. So, if you're not taking part in a clinical therapy with this substance, in a medical institution that is practicing this type of treatment or trials, it would be advisable to make sure your or your guide's source is trustworthy.

Moreover, when dealing with psychedelics, you become more aware of the energy that comes with the particular substance you consume. Some experienced users have even said they can feel the energy of the one who made the acid and the people that handled it before it got to them. Even if you don't have such a holistic approach to the experience, you can admit that it makes a difference if you were given LSD by a friendly, loving person or a nasty dealer.

As for toxicity, an LSD trip is as toxic as an aspirin, and this says a lot not only about its purity, but also about its general compatibility with the human organism.

19

THE SIMILARITIES AND DIFFERENCES BETWEEN LSD, PSILOCYBIN MUSHROOMS, MDMA & DMT

These are the four main candidates for psychedelic therapy today used in a few traditional clinics in medical environments by unauthorized guides and urban shamans that take you in nature or in a pleasant interior, and probably most of all in self-therapy by people who pursue self-development, self-healing, creative inspiration, or spiritual endeavors. Each is very different than the other, but all of them are used to treating the main mental conditions affecting our contemporary society: depression, anxiety, PTSD, and addiction. In this sense, one could notice the paradox of these truly helpful substances that are used under hiding and more often than not in party contexts where they are unconsciously abused, as well as the irony of being under the restrictment of the law.

Apart from magic mushrooms, which are the fruits of mother nature, the other three are chemical compounds synthesized in labs from a number of sources. This has a profoundly distinct effect on the nature of the trip, in which the natural medicinal substances inducing hallucinations, trance, or any other psychedelic experiences are said to come with a spirit guide. The sensation is as if the drug's spirit enters your being and gets a grip on you, guiding your journey and grounding you at the same time, although the feeling is sometimes so strong that it can become unbearable unless you release the control and thus free yourself.

With the magic mushrooms, this feeling, as if you sensed the spirit of the mushroom inside of you, is very strong, and depending on the type of fungi, it can be unpredictable, pushing you from one state to another, from one dimension of perception to the next. The visuals are organic, morphing one into the other, bringing on visions of the vegetal earth and creatures from our mythology. On the contrary, when taking an artificially synthesized compound, the sensation is very different, and the simplest way to describe it is more digital in appearance.

The LSD visuals are not as strong as with mushrooms or DMT. They seem to be an enhancement of reality, as hallucinations are almost none or not the hyper science-fiction type that you experience with DMT when travelling the worlds of planets or the visceral kind of shrooms. With LSD, you see the subtle definition of the matrix within the images of vibrations. In this, MDMA is unique as it lacks the visuals; you don't see mandalas or dragons, no supernatural beings, and not much transformations from the normal visual perception, just a better focus and overall clarity. It is worth mentioning that MDMA is neither a psychedelic nor an amphetamine but something in between.

Looking from a more generic point of view, we can say the trip on LSD is similar to that of one induced by the magic mushrooms, in terms of length and intensity, as well as the type of energy and rhythm it sustains. LSD is the most active and energetic of them all, keeping you alive and alert, indifferent of an uplifting or bad tripping vibe. DMT is the shortest, lasting only 15 minutes, compared to the few hours that you experience on any of the other three, depending on the dose. It's also the fastest to take effect, plunging you in hyperspace moments after administration, whereas the others take at least half an hour to start.

With DMT, although you have an awakened consciousness, the awareness of the space you find yourself in is completely lost as you get transported to completely surreal dimensions, while lying in some kind of immobile trance. Mushrooms can have such a profoundly grounding effect in high doses, incapacitating your motion and putting you in an introspective state where your travels are exclusively within.

LSD can turn out both ways; it can either send your attention within or make you literally jump and embrace reality when you find yourself in nature, igniting a different sense of perceiving the textures of grass and trees, as they breathe in fascinating visual expressions, feeling the fresh smell of flowers and the way all these senses interfere with one another. MDMA is also rather malleable, as on a high dose, you'd want to lie down and take the process within, but when taking less, you're left with enough energy to feel the love of the universe while walking around with few impediments.

LSD, DMT, MDMA, as well as magic mushrooms are psychotropic substances that alter the normal way in which you perceive reality by opening your perspective to see the depthness and multidimensionality. They all establish the connection with the intricate nature of the universe, with the wilderness of the world, and with your true self, enabling you to contain and experience the whole of your being and thus the complexity of life. As such, their after-effects and what is considered their healing potential are the senses of awareness and clarity of a more sustainable self-acceptance and self-confidence of meaning and, have the remarkable result of generating beneficial change in one's life.

MDMA differs from all in focusing its action on the emotional plane. As an effect, it induces the sensation of love, universal love. As a matter of fact, with MDMA it's the most powerful vibration. It transcends the being, making you feel an overwhelmingly dear emotion towards all the people that are important in your life, towards life itself, towards your surroundings and those that are immediately close to you. For this reason, MDMA is especially helpful when it comes to overcoming traumas, allowing you to accept and forgive, to express compassion towards your being and the others involved.

Concerning the chemical structure and the way it interacts with our brain, all these substances have a different means, but they all interfere with the levels of serotonin and dopamine. Despite all others, DMT also has a particular character, being a naturally occurring compound in the human body. They all increase interconnectivity in the brain, outlining the complex network of our thoughts by switching patterns that are usually in standby and inducing a state of happiness and self-meaning.

In terms of toxicity, even though a synthesized chemical, LSD is the least harmful compound, interfering with your organism at minimum, while the MDMA is the most toxic of our list.

20

THE FUTURE OF LSD

The further exploration of lysergic acid is strongly connected with the future research on consciousness. The study of consciousness, in the form of a veritable science field, emerged with the new psychedelic era. One of the main points of interest concerning the LSD experience is its huge potential in revealing more and more about human consciousness through the experience of different states of being and perceiving.

The pioneers of the 50's and 60's praised this miraculous compound, infusing its image with all their peace, freedom and love ideals, with a belief that reality is not what the constricting social system is teaching us but an infinite beyond. Today's followers of the past memorable cultural figures igniting the psychedelic revolution are actually scientists, continuing their work in a frame that has the power to clean the reputation of LSD and proclaim its transcending potential.

The traditional world of medicine and science as a whole is accepting the peculiarities of the psychedelic experience in all its intensity, its extraordinary insights in past lives, out-of-body journeys, shifts of states bordering mental psychosis or schizophrenia, and the whole palette that the new-age devotees call 'spiritual awakening'. This opens a most promising future in therapy for lysergic acid, and hopefully, the laws will become properly permissive to allow the growth of research and experimentation.

The rising interest in LSD coincides with a new revival of the spiritual movement that also began in the hippie period with the Western import of Eastern practices and their integration in processes of self-development. All these drives point to an acute crisis of the world today, a crisis of individuality, as well as one of the community, a necessity to contain the ancestral wisdom of our predecessors that held a special connection with nature and their true selves, while integrating it in the understanding and routine of modern society.

A strong need to rediscover the spiritual nature of life and reality is reflected in the enthusiasm that mystic materials present to an ever wider spectrum of population, like divination methods, tarot, astrology, numerology, and a variety of other old sciences that reappear in new forms. The culture of psychedelics, and of LSD implicitly, not only rides the same wave, but also offers a gateway to the source where all these answers can be found, along with the deeper insights of the universe that we don't even know how to address yet.

We can also discuss the influence that LSD, as well as other psychedelics, have on the trend of raving people that consume drugs recreationally at parties. Although LSD can be found on the list of party drugs, a veritable experience on lysergic acid is strong enough to produce a shift consciousness such as to pursue a path of awareness, where you create an addiction. One's behavior and attachments are profoundly transformed in a way that he compassionately accepts himself and the world in its entire complexity, the good along with the bad, and this makes a person much less vulnerable, more confident, and persevering on the track that he finds meaningful for his life. As a consequence, the use of LSD has the potential to stop the abuse of psychotropic substances, replacing it with a longing of further learning and discovery.

The microdosing of LSD seems to be more and more appealing, and again, it fits perfectly on the typology of today's society. Even though the practice does not reach the level of mysticism that those on a spiritual path might be looking for, it is nonetheless a clean and efficient therapeutic means through which people can relieve their anxiety and depression, their day to day pressure, by creating a new paradigm of perceiving reality and structuring their lives towards well-being. As it appears, the future of LSD seems prolific in many directions, and this is mostly because its intricate character matches the social diversity of the contemporary man and therefore offers a solution for a variety of its modern and not so modern needs.

The rising number of urban guides that organize private, hidden therapeutic sessions with LSD is proof of acid's incredible effects, as is its use in self-exploratory and self-treatment pursuits. More than anything, it shows that people trust the substance above the therapist, enough to bypass the law, as well as the instated fear of its dangerous potential. Not to say that these underground guides are not reliable modern shamans, because most of them are doing it as they truly believe in its positive effects and consider their mission and vocation to share these beautiful experiences with others in need.

The money they receive for this service couldn't stand for a sufficient reason in this case, because they have to go through an ordeal to hide their profession and construct a different clandestine persona. If you read through the internet, you can find stories of such guides, inquiries that, of course, keep their identity secret, and discover that they are all normal people. They're not new-age hippies going to festivals, wearing tribal outfits, and promoting enlightenment; on the contrary, they're dressed in suits and spend their days in offices like the majority of us.

LSD is, for them, a means to evolve their beings. Even though they don't give acid to people at a campfire doing incantations, they know well enough how to show respect to the substance and to ensure the perfect set and setting, so their sessions are the equivalent of modern rituals, taken with the precaution of concealment. Their clients are normal people, taking their chances because they believe in the testimonies of people that had taken it before and have received precious insights that helped them change their lives for the better.

As it's seen, LSD is gaining a good reputation and credibility on the streets, not only used recreationally but therapeutically, and without the aid of legal or medical institutions, without too much research or writing available that could establish its trustworthy image, with only word of mouth and the belief in people's stories. In this line of thought, LSD seems to have a promising future independent of conventional mainstream efforts in this direction.

21
LSD - THE PSYCHEDELIC REMEDY OF THE MODERN MAN

If you are looking to start psychedelic therapy, LSD appears as the substance that's most friendly to begin with. It's not controllable. You have to release control so as not to be trapped in a loop and unable to take advantage of the benefits of the experience, but it is introducing you to other dimensions of thought, distorting the vision of reality without exhibiting a different existence altogether. The trip lies in the discovery of different new possibilities, lying at hand, to experience the very world we live in. The lack of strong hallucinations gives the feeling that what you see is not in fact a distortion, but an enhancement.

This book is not meant to be promotional material for LSD; rather, its purpose is to present and explain, as factually as possible, the fascination and praise that is continually growing around this psychedelic substance. The image of a drug that has the potential of abuse doesn't stand so firmly against the myriads of positive enlightening testimonials or against the psychedelic nature of LSD. Considering that an abusive user would only have part of bad trips, one would have virtually no reason to engage in such a way of consumption. The LSD journeys are such powerful, transformational experiences that is actually hard to believe that a human being can take one after the other, the way it happens with drugs that offer instant relief or glimpse of ecstasy, like amphetamines or recreational drugs.

One of the most important aspects when taking acid, or any other psychedelic, is the intention that you start with. This is an essential part of the inner setting that one has to prepare before the actual experience. The intention gives the direction of the whole journey, and if it is healing a past trauma or discovering your own spirituality, that is where LSD will take you.

Any intention that is not compatible with your being or with the nature of this substance will be impeded from the beginning and gifted with a bad trip. Reading and hearing what people have to say about it, you may notice that the ones that took acid just to have more fun but had a horrific bad trip are mentioning it as the sole experience they had on LSD. This is very different than reliving past tormenting issues or the confrontations with your own darkside that one should expect when pursuing a process of healing traumas, because in these cases, the experience is assumed from the start, and the whole journey is therapy on fast forward. Thus, LSD is the modern equivalent of the ancient trance plant medicines, a substance to fit and treat the most troubling problems of the modern man.

PART III

THE BEGINNERS INTRODUCTORY GUIDE TO DMT

PSYCHEDELICS AND THE DIMETHYLTRYPTAMINE MOLECULE: PSYCHEDELIC CURIOSITY

It may be that DMT makes us able to perceive what the physicist call "dark matter" - the 95 per cent of the universe's mass that is know to exist but that at present remains invisible to our senses and instruments.

— Graham Hancock

22
A PORTAL TO THE MULTIVERSE WITHIN

The journey on DMT takes you to distant places that seem to be the point of intersection of multiple worlds. You may consider the experience to be a very personal one, a descent into your inner world and the discovery of the scenarios and creatures that populate it. But what people who took DMT describe, although unique for each individual in certain aspects, contains to many similarities to disregard the collective nature of this hallucinogenic experience.

Set yourself free of preconceptions, and if this is a hard thing to do nowadays, know that, in what concerns DMT, spirituality as well as science are on the same page. Take a step forward towards accepting and containing all of yourself, all that is. Let this book be your guide into the mysteries of this miraculous compound, and follow it to discover the profound and complex potential of your own consciousness.

23

ENTERING THE PARADOX

The effect of DMT is hard to describe in metaphors, hyperboles, oxymorons and similes because it is the expression of the essential paradox of life. As it's been portrayed, DMT reveals the matrix of reality and plunges you into the multiverse, into the vast infinite dimensional realm of parallel realities. Neither perception nor clarity of mind are distorted but heightened.

What each understands from this unearthly endeavor is, though, mostly personal. Some have healed past traumas, others have overcome addictions and great fears, most have faced their denials and understood why their lives unrolled the way they did and what their purpose in this existence is now. What is common for all reports from users is the state of enlightenment and the unbelievable expansion of consciousness.

24

A GATE TO ANOTHER WORLD

DMT is an omnipresent molecule, embedded in the chemical structure of virtually all living organisms. If you can imagine that this outstanding compound that has the potential of offering you the experience of infinite lifetimes in just a few minutes, is extractable from mere grass then you can start to grasp its magic. As the saying goes, the greatest treasures of the world are hidden under your eyes, so take a step out and a better look at your lawn. Look at the flowers, the trees, the ants in the ground and the birds in the sky. Look at your dog, at the mosquito you just squashed, look at yourself. DMT is everywhere you look.

Of course dimethyltryptamine is not the only recurrent substance in both plants and animals, but for now, no other one has been found to provoke such a mind-blowing and life-changing effect when consumed. No other one to reveal the substance of life, the intricate connection bonding space and time and all living things. Could it be that DMT's pervasive nature is signaling us that we are indeed all one, a single united consciousness? Can DMT tackle the contemporary problem of singularity?

The syntagm that became the stamp to define this incredible compound, 'the spirit molecule' is referring to the spiritual dimension that DMT awakens, the connection with a higher force, with the prime source of energy. By igniting a complete sense of awareness, it reveals the universal blueprint of life. Yet, this is not schematic knowledge that can be translated in words or scientific terms, we don't have the proper concepts in order to explain this type of information.

It goes beyond the characters and events you meet during the trip, and can only be contained by the state of spirit that's induced in you, because if you were to analyze the mind-boggling endeavors that people recount having after consuming DMT, you would be inquiring the immense basin of archetypal stories that mankind ever imagined. But the essential aspect is that these fairytale stories, even though resembling hallucinations or dreams, were vividly experienced, with an awakened mind, clear, utterly attentive and perceptive, with all the senses heightened and feeling completely new sensations.

This type of sensitivity is unprecedented not only in all first-time users but also in all human experience in the course of history. It could be assimilated as a most powerful religious experience, or in modern terms, as a true spiritual awakening, but both these concepts are not extensive enough to contain what one lives when taking DMT. And this is mainly because the DMT trip feels much more real than both, it's as if you were sensing multiple dimensions of reality that have not been addressed by any of the literature that's been generated by humans till the present moment.

Moreover, it's as if you were sensing this multiverse with senses that you couldn't have dreamed of possessing, while totally unable to define the experience using the rational predicaments we are used to. The DMT journey is therefore a complex phenomenon that surpasses and defies the scientific laws and religious scriptures.

Nonetheless, this new wave of consciousness is gaining momentum with more and more adepts, and gradually yet rapidly building around it a new narrative. This is the narrative of the new men. In this line of thought, can we talk about the DMT culture in terms of a new religion? Even if we are merely taking the first steps in this next generation of thinking and perceiving reality, we might as well call it that.

The most important change that this DMT culture is bringing to our consciousness is the bridging of religion and science, the two disciplines that have guided human evolution to where we are now, while being in constant conflict with each other. We've already sketched the spiritual dimension that you are submerged in when doing DMT, but what is more spectacular is that it describes the key concepts that quantum physics is working with.

During the DMT trip you have the sensation that time and space warp in a continuum dimension, or in other words, that there is no past or future but an eternal present and that space is infinite. Moreover, this type of environment grants you the ability to be everywhere in this very moment, the same way in which quantum physics explains that the laws of the microcosmos allow the molecules to be in more places in the same time. In this sense, you could say that DMT is actually bending the structure and ordinary dynamics of your mind in order to accept the existence of multiple layers of reality and an infinite potential of manifestation. Simply said, this would mean to accept the inherent paradox of life.

25

EXPERIENCING DEATH

DMT has been associated with the concept and experience of death in many ways, starting with the idea that became a meme, stating that DMT is produced by the body at the moment of death, which is a plausible and provocative speculation, but not yet a proven fact.

This concept has been pushed extensively since the launch of 'The spirit molecule' book and documentary, where Dr. Rick Strassman, its author, is suggesting that this compound may be released by our bodies when entering special states of consciousness like meditation, sleep, trance or death. Furthermore, this movie, as well as the research in this subject, have inquired the individual experiences of different people who confessed their out-of-body journeys on DMT were indeed, feeling as if they had died.

The DMT trip propels your consciousness out of the ordinary presence, out of your body, cutting the connection with the material dimension. The trance that you enter, although extremely short, is enrapturing you in a completely different state of being, where your perception is not anymore guided by your five senses, but from a central point within your being, by the inner sense of awareness.

The worlds that you travel through are perceived in a totally different manner because you are sensing everything as raw as it is, unobstructed by the inherent limitations of our five senses, and neither by the predetermined understanding of our minds. As such, DMT takes you in an exploration of new territories, in which you find yourself a new being, using new instruments of guidance. Of course, in a realm where space and time are superfluous, where the entire spectrum of vision is distorted and populated with dream-like visions, the feeling that you are not anymore on this planet, becomes more than reasonable.

The strong sense of detachment from the physical plane, amplified by the inability to receive stimuli from the physical reality while you are submerged in the inner journey, is contributing substantially to the impression that you've just died.

But there are other substances that induce a similar detachment, ketamine is one of the synthetic compounds that present such an effect, and there's also a number of plant medicines that fall into the same category, among which are peyote, iboga or psychedelic mushrooms. They're not however associated with death as much as DMT is.

This is due to DMT's modus operandi, the dynamic through which it cuts your connections to materiality not only by pausing your senses of orientation, but also by collapsing your entire mental structure, your ego. This is the essential shock that one goes through and that creates the powerful illusion of dying. By dissolving your identity, DMT is in fact erasing what you are used to calling you, and the great surprise is that without an identity, your consciousness continues to exist. This occurrence, termed as 'ego death' has been intensively inquired as it has important implications from philosophical as well as scientific points of view, starting with the question of what exactly is consciousness, and if there is life after death.

Most of the people that took DMT report coming back from this presumed death, with a feeling of an intense spiritual awakening that left them with the comforting sensation that life may continue after we die. But the conviction that the conscious ego will dwell further than our flesh is apparently nothing more than a whimsical hope. Nonetheless, DMT proves that our consciousness is not bounded by our ego and that our sense of awareness does not depend upon our individuality.

DMT tackles this fundamental question of humanity, what happens after we die, a problem that men have tried to get a vision of through all possible means, that has been interpreted by religion, philosophy and science in multiple scenarios. What's all the more spectacular is that the DMT trip, like the near-death experiences, produces very similar visions. People recount having the same sense of detachment from their bodies, seeing a tunnel that sweeps them into a bright white light, and taking them to dreamlike realms where they met entities of light, which the more religious of them describe as saints.

So, it seems reasonable that dimethyltryptamine is associated with death and furthermore it can be a unique way in which you can confront your fear of death. But is it actually threatening your life? Can DMT induce death? The answer is no. The quantity of substance that is enough to produce one very strong trip, is far from endangering your health. What the famous psychonaut Terence Mckenna had to say about this issue was that death can occur in a DMT experience, only if 'death by astonishment' is possible.

26

A BRIEF HISTORY OF DMT USE

The use of trance medicinal plants containing DMT goes far back down our historic timeline than the actual synthesization of the compound by modern chemists. Its original use was traced to South America, but considering that it was primarily employed by tribal cultures that had no other means to register their knowledge and history but through oral communication, we actually have no certainty that DMT based plants were not consumed in other parts of the world as well.

The well-known Amazonian hallucinogenic brew Ayahuasca, is made from the leaves of the Chacruna plant, Psychotria Viridis, or the Chagropanga plant, Diplopterys Cabrerana, that contain high concentrations of DMT, combined with the Banisteriopsis Caapi vine, which brings to the whole compound a most necessary addition.

The tropical vine is included in the drink to prolong the trance effect because it contains harmine, a substance that inhibits the breakdown of the dimethyltryptamine by our digestive system. This explains why the Ayahuasca trance takes as long as eight to nine hours, compared with the DMT trip, which is about fifteen minutes, of which the highest state lasts for only five. This will be more clearly explained in the next chapter when we'll be discussing the chemical processes occurring in the body with the intake of this compound.

It's important to remember that Amazonian cultures knew the way DMT worked long before it became popular among modern civilization. The earliest records of the traditional use of DMT containing plants date from the 8th century when it was apparently utilized to produce psychoactive snuffs, as the cohoba for example, made from the seeds of Anadenanthera Peregrina.

But even in South America, Ayahuasca was restricted to tribal cultures as it caught the interest of the wider public and started to spread when the rubber industry exploded in the Amazon. It opened a door through which civilization entered the jungle and traditional knowledge, in exchange, stepped in the urban environment.

The enthusiasm with the medicine brew was so big that it spawned an entire religion, a series of Ayahuasca cults appearing in Brazil, merging the traditional beliefs of the Amazons with the Brazilian cosmology and Catholicism. The first Ayahuasca religion, Santo Daime, was founded in 1930, and after the seventies it started to expand to other continents, today is recognized as an established spiritual cult that is permitted to use its main Ayahuasca ritual in many countries of the world.

The chemical DMT was first discovered and synthesized in 1931 by Richard Manske, a Canadian chemist, but at that moment nothing else was known about this compound. Then in 1946, Oswaldo Goncalves de Lima, a microbiologist, found that DMT is naturally occurring in plants. But it wasn't until ten years later, in 1956, that Stephen Szara made it known of the psychoactive effects of the substance.

The Hungarian chemist and psychiatrist became familiar with DMT during his travels to South America where he participated in traditional religious ceremonies with plant medicine and remained fascinated. He then extracted DMT from the Mimosa Hostilis plant and injected himself with the compound intramuscularly, and his discoveries spawned the Western curiosity regarding this mind-altering substance and the medicinal and hallucinogenic cultures of the Amazon.

In 1965 Franzen and Gross discovered that DMT was to be found in the urine and blood of humans. This finding, sent them on a misleading route, as they suspected the occurrence of DMT within our bodies was related to mental imbalances such as schizophrenia. The explanation was that this condition may be the effect of a metabolic error of the human body, which produced this type of hallucinogen and thus sickened the brain.

Of course, the studies produced no hard evidence to link dimethyltryptamine with the respective mental condition, but fortunately it triggered the scientific interest towards the amazing effects on consciousness and the extraordinary ways in which it interacts with the normal dynamics of the brain.

The ecstatic hippie period of the 60's and 70's provided a fertile context for the research into the effects of DMT, and a great number of papers were produced by prominent figures of the time like Alan Watts and Timothy Leary, a body of work that more than anything else, marked the first steps into the modern study of consciousness. The set back came in 1970 when the Controlled Substances Act was to pause any further research into DMT, or other psychedelic substances, in USA as well as Europe.

Another wave of recognition was ignited by Terence Mckenna who popularized his enthusiasm for DMT's incredible potential around the 80's and 90's, when he extensively explored and documented the substance, while also traveling to get to know its Amazonian origins and the traditional manners in which indigenous people used it.

It took thirty years for the story of DMT to come back to the public eye, but this time it was going to hit the front pages and become a mainstream phenomenon. It all happened in the 90's when Rick Strassman started to research further the effects that hallucinogens produce in our brains, enhancing perception, and essentially expanding our consciousness. After delivering a number of studies on the subjective response to this type of substance in different individuals, including the outputs of different doses, in the year 2000 he published 'The Spirit Molecule', a book that is still the main reference in any discussion about DMT.

The book was followed by a documentary, in 2010, that the director Mitch Schultz did in collaboration with Dr. Strassman, and which paved the way for an entire culture surrounding the DMT phenomenon. DMT was gaining adepts not only among the scientists, philosophers or those concerned with researching consciousness but building a much greater audience.

'The spirit molecule' became the famous nickname of dimethyltryptamine, and this indicated another level of public awareness in regards to this compound that was known earlier in the sixties as 'the businessman's trip' due to its short time effect and lack of aftereffects when coming back. Its new label marked DMT's upgrading from a drug substance to a consciousness expanding compound.

Extensive research into DMT was produced also by the famous chemists Alexander and Anna Shulgin, who have synthesized, experimented with and documented most of the psychotropic substances that are now illegally used, as well as legally studied and employed in therapy worldwide. 'Tihkal' is the name of their publication in which they talk about the effects of tryptamines when smoked or consumed orally in different dosages.

Since it became known all over the world, DMT is gaining more and more popularity, due to the scientific interest that it presents and the studies that follow, in the quest of exploring its potential use in therapy as well as an instrument to indulge into the new discipline of consciousness. The grand-scale familiarity and usage of dimethyltryptamine is owed in part to its fairly easy process of extraction, which makes it an available activity to anyone with little chemistry know-how, although it still is a Schedule 1 substance from a legal point of view.

27

CHEMISTRY, PHARMACOLOGY & EFFECTS

DMT, or N, N-dimethyltryptamine is an endogenous indole alkaloid found widely in plants and animals, pertaining to the class of tryptamines, as its analogous compounds 5-hydroxy-DMT and 5-methoxy-DMT. Its chemical structure resembles those of serotonin and melatonin, as well as other hallucinogenic substances.

DMT is said to occur naturally as a by-product of our bodies and although there is not sufficient proof to clearly determine this, it's been discovered within our bodies in enough concentrations to suggest it does have a specific role. According to the well-known myth concerning the inherent production of DMT by our bodies, it is supposedly generated by the pineal gland. There's insufficient evidence to state this as a fact in humans, but DMT has been found in the pineal gland of rats.

DMT's synthesis within our bodies starts from tryptophan that becomes tryptamine and then with the action of INMT (indolethylamine-N-methyltransferase), N-methyltryptamine is created, which is finally catalyzed into DMT. INMT is mostly found in the thyroid, lungs and adrenal gland, as well as in the pineal gland, although other areas of the brain are scarce in this compound.

The trick is that these areas that are fertile for the production of DMT, are also containing the necessary enzymes that can break it down and suppress its absorption into the bloodstream. These MAO-A, monoamine oxidase A, act very rapidly, as such any trace of DMT disappears from the blood in less than an hour.

Studies have found that the main action of DMT is upon the serotonin receptors, more precisely on the 5-HT2A receptor. Researching further, it has been indicated that DMT also affects dopamine and sigma-1 receptors. Inquiring its bonding to sigma-1 receptor may bring significant clues in explaining the role of the naturally occurring DMT, otherwise the mystery of why our bodies produce this substance prevails over all assumptions.

The sigma-1, receptor which is detected throughout our bodies, is ensuring that our cells don't die in low oxygen situations, whereof this can be the basis of the theory that DMT is generated in abundance when we die in a desperate attempt to resurrect the dying cells. In this line of thought, the body appears to give itself an overdose of DMT in order to survive, providing us with the psychedelic experience as collateral. This would explain why a lot of subjects who have experienced near-death reported mystical encounters, a state of detachment and profound spiritual awareness.

The effects are wide ranging, starting from a generally uplifting sensation that can be described as euphoria of the mind, body and heart. In this sense, it should be stated that it accelerates the heart rate, and generally, this is the down-side in terms of negative side-effects.

On a physical level, DMT induces a sense of spatial disorientation, and with the detachment from the body comes as well a disruption in sensing temperature, and distortion of gravity, one can feel as light as a feather and be propelled light-years away in a matter of fractions of seconds.

As for the mental effects, there are a plethora of symptoms, from the ego death that we've discussed earlier, to cognitive euphoria and a substantial improvement of the analytical function, to delusion and deja-vu sensations. A state of mindfulness is induced, where the memory of individuality disappears, and in this state, novelty is welcomed and appreciated as it's bringing along the total refresh of consciousness.

Mind capacity is essentially expanded such as to contain multiple streams of thought in a dynamic structure that flows freely in the absence of time and space. In a bad trip all these aspects can be reversed in anxiety and paranoia when the actual trip cannot be contained as a temporary experience and is taken with the fear of death, surpassing the enthusiasm of the new.

The sense of sight is enhanced in a most amazing manner with the image flipping, melting and morphing in a symmetrical and repetitive pattern, with a color acuity that makes everything glow. The vision is somewhere in between digital and organic, where the perfect geometry of sharp angles collapses in round corners and soft edges, only to shift again in a complex structure. On the other hand, the sense of hearing is not affected at such extents, it is merely enhanced to a more ample set of vibrations, but this is rather occurring at the end of the DMT trip.

The hallucinatory effect can manifest in a myriad of ways, but certain phenomenons are similar for every user. Be it internal or external, the visions are autonomous and interactive, lucid and transcendental, be it of spiritual, fantasy or science-fiction nature. What's most significant though from a therapeutic point of view, are the transpersonal effects, from the erasing of identity to an enhanced perception of self-meaning, understanding the existential purpose and the mechanics of consciousness, while experiencing a sense of unity and interconnectivity with everything there is.

There are a few stages that the DMT trip goes through, from the on-set that starts with an enhancement in vision and mental penetration, the forming of geometrical patterns and crackling or high pitched sounds. After breaking through you find yourself in a sort of waiting room or rather waiting channel, as it seems more like a tunnel with rapidly shifting geometry, through which you are pushed with the speed of light until the other side.

That is where you find the parallel realities populated with the collective archetypes enriched with your own unconscious imagery. It is there where you experience the peak of your transformational journey, meeting the entities and exploring cosmic landscapes. From this point the coming back is as if you're gradually sucked away from that dimension, further and further until you reach Earth again, in which time the realms you've traveled to along with the memory itself of this experience, quickly dissipates. The previous state of presence in the parallel multiverse dies out after about ten minutes, and along with it, the visions disappear as well. The trip leaves you in a state of excitement and awe, a high that you can feel in the body for almost an hour after.

28

PROPER DMT CONSUMPTION

As with everything in our modern speedy age, we wish for everything that we do to take as a short while as possible, in a most simple manner and to leave us fresh enough to return to work, tasks, friends or whatever routine we have. For this reason 'the businessman's trip' was perfect in so many ways. It takes just a couple of minutes to take your stash of DMT crystals out of your pocket and into the pipe, heat it, inhale the vapors and in no time you are catapulted in other dimensions.

The effect takes off in less than a second. The single thing you have to take care of is your setting, you can't do it standing the way you smoke your cigarette in a break, and you wouldn't want your colleagues to watch you trippin'. But other than that, in just twenty minutes from the moment you took the first deep breath in, you'll be as fresh as before, at least.

Thus, you can skip your lunch break and use it to travel light miles away, visit infinite worlds and taste eternity. Of course this mind-blowing experience would require some time to relax and contain the enormous amount of information you've just received. But nonetheless, all this visionary trance is diluted in great proportion in the few moments it takes for you to come down from the peak of the trip to the three-dimensional reality, just like the dream evaporates from your memory when you open your eyes.

There's only fragments that stay with you, glimpses to remind you that indeed you went away, and it wasn't all just your vivid imagination. There's no aftereffect of dizziness, confusion or physical impairment to stop you from getting back to whatever you've been doing before, so nobody can notice anything suspect with you, or maybe just a more clear, active, present and enthusiastic attitude, but in this case, you could just blame it on the double shot espresso you just had.

29

PROPER PREPARATION

Approaching this mysterious substance in the manner described above is appropriate only for the experienced users that are familiar with the substance, with the journey and are able to grasp and contain the miraculous experience with clarity and awareness. Otherwise, the recreational consumption of DMT could be a lack of respect towards the immense potential of knowledge this molecule can offer you.

Its Amazonian counterpart is taken in a complex ritual that prepares your body, but most of all, your mind, to be able to smoothly navigate the cosmic waters and integrate the gifts of this voyage in a most helpful manner.

Ayahuasca is foremost a medicine and the attitude of the indigenous people towards consuming the plant brew is accordingly, they are searching for remedies, for purifying their spirits and material bodies as well, for enlightenment and precious insights from other spirit entities they meet during the trance.

To accomplish this, a special state of being is requested and you need to be in tune, open and respectful. As such, a particular diet is recommended to cleanse your system and allow the substance to pass gently, ease the purification work of the body to let the spiritual experience to occur with grace and no impediments. Extra rituals with different purgative plants are usually performed before the Ayahuasca ceremony, like tobacco tea that makes you release the toxins out of your body through vomiting, or using an even more powerful compound, as the venom of the Cambo frog that has the same purpose and a much powerful effect.

Of course these procedures are necessary because the Amazonian concoct activates through your digestive system and the more cluttered it is, the harder for the medicine to make its way. The whole hallucinogenic trance is affected by the hops and blockages which are in return reflected in not so pleasant visions.

This is because, as we all know by now, everything within us is connected, it's just that we are not yet able to translate this properly, so an upset bowel can be seen as a furious dragon and, while caught up in distant unknown worlds, you may just miss it and confuse it for what it is not.

In the case of DMT that needs no digestion to take effect inside your body and mind, this type of preparation becomes superfluous. However, what 'the businessman' bypasses in the whole process is that the period of physical preparation constitutes a chance to prepare your consciousness for the leap of faith that DMT, as Ayahuasca, offers.

It represents a time in which you concentrate your full awareness on freeing old unbalanced mind-patterns and setting out in the journey with clear intentions. The toxins in your body make your brain foggy and confused which may induce anxiety, fear and miss-judgment, for which reasons the Amazonians use purging on a regular basis. You could say it's almost like plucking the weeds and preparing the soil to be fertile enough to nurture and grow the new seeds you're about to plant.

Knowing the stages of this process that the South Americans perfected in a very long time of constant work with the plant medicine, can give you an idea about the manner in which you should approach any substance that has the potential of a psychotropic healing experience. So, unless you're the type of businessman that devotedly practices his daily transcendental meditation and are therefore able to enter a mindful state by the clap of your hands, it would be recommended to take some time off and prepare yourself a ritualic setting of the interior and exterior space before you indulge in inhaling DMT.

30

INSTRUMENTS & TECHNIQUES

DMT in the form of crystals can be smoked or vaporized, but either way it is highly important for the flame not to touch the compound such as not to lose its potency in the air before it gets in your lungs.

You can use a freebase pipe, or meth pipe, in which case you put the crystals directly in the bulb, then heat up the glass to vaporize the substance and inhale it. Keep the smoke in for 10-20 seconds, then breathe out and repeat the process. A more efficient instrument is the glass vapor genie that practically ensures you there's no loss of DMT, in the heating or burning and that it all gets inside your system.

The most common way to consume DMT is the sandwich method, in which you place the DMT crystals in between the leaves of a plant, be it marijuana or another plant and put it in a pipe or a bong. Proceeding in this manner will necessitate much more attention as you have to be careful to merely heat the upper leaves and not burn them. It's the simplest method when you don't have other more adequate equipment, but it leaves room for so many errors that you will have to be prepared with extra DMT material to refill in order to truly get a breakthrough. What you can do to increase the efficiency is to create a gravity bong, so as to pile up the smoke inside and take a full inhalation at the end.

Another more sophisticated process is to enhance the plant leaves with DMT, or in simpler words, to infuse the inactive plant with a DMT solution, and afterward smoke it. This is done by immersing the DMT and plant in a solvent, be it isopropyl alcohol, butane or acetone, leave it and wait patiently for a few days till the solvent evaporates, and only afterward consume it. This is very similar to the substance that goes by the name changa, but this plant mix uses an addition of a MAOI containing herb that prolongs the experience. Plants like blue Lotus, Passionflower or Caapi are used, but as the testimonials report, even though the effect goes on for a considerable longer period, the high is substantially less strong.

Important Tip

Either way you choose, there's one essential aspect that you have to remember and this is advice from experienced users, something Terence Mckenna repeated with each and every occasion. When you feel you're about to take off, take one more big inhalation. That and only that will do the job. Otherwise you'd just get a glimpse of the other unearthly worlds, a mere check out from the window and not have enough propulsion to fly off this planet.

This is a mistake most first time users make when they don't have proper guidance. If you don't do it in the right time, which is right away, then you will have to wait for a while for MAO-A to clear out of your system. Otherwise the DMT you consume will be immediately broken down without any chance of transforming into the miraculous voyage you're so eagerly expecting.

Extraction

Most common plants out of which DMT is extracted are the root barks of Acacia Confusa or Mimosa Hostilis, although there is a great number of other herbs that can be used. The variety of extraction methods are able to suit any level of chemistry knowledge. The simplest is to take the grounded plant matter and immerse it into a base solution, usually sodium hydroxide, which literally dissolves the plant and leaves the DMT molecules floating in the liquid.

To separate the DMT, a non-polar solvent is added in order to attract the non-polar DMT molecules out of the polar base you've just used. The non-polar solvent, now containing the DMT molecules, separates itself in a different layer and can be easily siphoned out of the base solution. In the end, through evaporation or freezing, you can liberate the DMT molecules out of the solvent, leaving you with the crystals that are ready to be heated and inhaled.

31
ENTERING THE HALLWAY OF ALL POSSIBLE REALITIES

Each DMT journey is unique not only from one individual to another, but also the trips of the same person greatly differ from each other. You can say it is like entering another door each time you take this substance, which can be said as well about other psychedelics, but in the case of DMT the endeavor is so incredible that it seems like completely distinct lifetimes altogether. You feel like a different entity each time around.

In all instances you experience the multiverse, the infinite parallel realities merging into each other, morphing in unimaginable forms and colors, in patterns that dissipate and rearrange constantly at high speeds, in front of your very eyes and throughout your body. You feel you are one with everything that is occurring, not only participating but existing in each and every geometric frame, dissolving with it and transforming into something else. And everything goes on indefinitely, all over the cosmos.

In these completely unknown and spectacular worlds where DMT takes you, you most curiously feel at home, for they're all entangled with our common reality, there's no sensation of rupture, it is all but one grand existence. This phenomenon fills you with a feeling of sacredness, with the impression that you are experiencing the very essence of life in a context much bigger than life itself.

It is therefore the spiritual awakening to a grander awareness in which you could literally say that you are meeting all virtual gods and most of all the god within. The sensation is that there is no difference between you and these sanctified entities, you are one of them. You are living the eternity in the infinity of space, and nothing gives off the suspicion of an illusion, instead it seems much more real than the reality we are accustomed to. You are being detached from your body, your senses, your memories, your entire self, and continuing to sense and understand through your consciousness.

In these distant realms you meet with different light entities that most often than not, welcome you with warmth and loving vibrations to their worlds, showing you around and inviting you to get a taste of the infinite. They are the most curious characters that not even your dreams have shown something similar.

They come in a variety of sizes and shapes, they sometimes have strawberry heads and machine like bodies, much like the well-known syntagm that Mckenna was using to describe his guides, the 'self-transforming machine elves'. There's always this combination between something digital and something organic, yet each time a slightly distinct god-like creature appearing in sight.

Even though it may not be of the same flesh and blood we're familiar with, it's nonetheless more real than our own bodies that we've just left behind. In this context, with you not having a body to structure your visible image in this multiverse, you may be wondering how do you look like for them. Maybe you're not wearing your usual humanoid cloak, maybe you also have an unbelievably wild and miraculous form just like them.

These friendly entities are your guides in the journey and besides giving you an unforgettable ride, they also work on your light body, giving you precious existential advice that has the potential of turning your life around. This is why most users confess they consume DMT for its therapeutic properties because they come back from their trips endorsed with powerful knowledge on what is good and meaningful for them.

Most DMT reports account for the meeting of a female or a male guide, a voice or even a character that leads them in their journeys. These guides are showing them the grand potential that lies within each, how to tap into this source of energy and use it for their own benefit, as well as for the greater good of humanity and life throughout the universes.

The interesting fact is that men usually encounter the female voice, and women the male's, which takes us to Carl Jung's theories of soul, who states that each man's soul is the Anima, the female within him, and each woman's soul is the Animus, the male within her. There's more connections between the DMT voyage and Jung's visions, for he talks extensively about the realm of the collective unconscious where all the figures that have ever populated the imagination and mythology of humankind, are gathered.

Whereof the dimensions that DMT discloses seem to be exactly that, with the only correction that the machine-like entities are nowhere to be found in the history of human thoughts and fantasies, they surpass all philosophies, religions and fairytales. In this sense, we may say that the DMT trip immerses us in collective universal consciousness of infinitely greater extents than our human unconscious.

32

DMT VS OTHER PSYCHEDELICS

Continuing the subject discussed just above concerning the realms one visits and entities one encounters during the DMT journey, we may start comparing it with its South American counterpart with which it shares most similarities, the Ayahuasca brew. The Amazonian plant medicine, in fact, draws much closer to Jung's theories in that it discloses precisely the fairytale lands of dreams and the archetypes that we got to know from fairytales, myths and other stories of that type.

For once, the Ayahuasca is known to echo the spirit of Mother Earth that comes embodied in a huge anaconda snake, a dragon-like appearance that seems to be the guide of the inner journey. The other spirits one meets during the eight hour voyage are all in one way or other familiar faces, presenting similitudes with something we've always known deep inside.

Although it is an extraordinary experience, the resemblances connect us with something from our memory, thus with our individuality and the collective individuality of humankind. For this reason, the whole journey is a very personal one, which brings forth the fears and anxieties tormenting the soul. On the contrary, with DMT, everything is so spectacularly new that you don't get the chance to sense fear, except the fear of novelty, of the unknown, of astonishment, not inner conflicts.

This also means that from a therapeutic point of view, the Amazonian plant medicine presents itself as a more efficient healer because it works directly with your problems. The anaconda travels within your being and spits out the blockages, the unresolved tensions, the sickness, cleansing your entity in its way out.

The duration of the whole experience is important in this aspect as well, as DMT is way shorter. We must also address the action upon the body: while DMT seems to have no physical effect, Ayahuasca makes you purge out all the accumulated toxins. The Curanderos of South America are praising specifically this property of the brew, putting higher importance on the purge than the visions it reveals, for the cleansing process is actually the healing one.

Going further, we may classify between the organic psychedelics and the synthesized substances, and present the fact that compounds as magic mushrooms, Ayahuasca, Iboga, Peyote, although very different from each other, they all come with a spirit guide that has origins in the nature of our planet, a spirit that you most definitely feel vibrating within you.

On the contrary, DMT, much like LSD are very different in this aspect, calling on entities that seem out of this realm, and often coming with no other guidance than your own consciousness. The senses of perception are very different especially because of the nature of the substance, wherein the synthesized compounds bring forth a more digital visualization of reality, resembling the structure of our modern culture and current imagery.

There are no 'self-transforming machine elves' in the magic mushroom trip unless you bring them in from your past DMT journey. In the DMT trip the digital and organic elements combine in one whole image of reality, and this seems to be a more truthful vision of reality as one unified consciousness field. The more we explore these other dimensions, the more we co-create, the more borders and differences between these realities melt and merge.

The main aspects that separate DMT from all the others and make it absolutely unreal, is the great potency and incredibly short duration. One LSD trip takes about 3-4 hours, a stronger magic mushroom experience can last 6-7 hours, whereas the journey on Ayahuasca or Peyote is 8-9 hours long, and an Iboga session can keep you in trance for more than 12 hours. In this context, the DMT journey seems to compress a whole universe in just one dot, the essence.

It resembles only one other compound and that is Salvia Divinorum, which as well takes off instantly and is over after 5-10 minutes. Unlike DMT, though, this type of sage is usually said to bring horrific visions of a distorted reality and the sense of detachment from your body. The physical plane is replaced with the disfiguration of the carnal and material informs that you not only you see but also feel.

There is no other psychotropic substance to catapult you out of this planet like DMT, to infuse you with exclusively novel information and sensations, to bridge unknown realities with a warm and peaceful welcoming. Of course this makes the journey more of an exploratory one than a therapeutic enterprise because it occupies your consciousness with a state of awe instead of pointing it towards the problems within your own body and psyche, which need your attention.

It directs your awareness outwards instead of inwards as the psychedelics do. You don't get to consciously confront your troubles because you simply forget about all of them, along with everything else related to your material existence. The therapy nonetheless happens in the background and with your conscious effort only after the trip is over. That is to say that it does take more energy and concentration to understand the teachings that you've received in your journey and implement the necessary changes in your daily life and in this physical reality.

On the opposite side though, the longer trips on Ayahuasca, Peyote and even LSD put you in front of your issues and you are supposed to resolve them during the trip. Most emotional or psychological blockages have to be dealt with at the beginning of the journey such as to smoothly take off and not get stuck in a loop. For this reason, the DMT interstellar voyages are generally much more peaceful and there's less potential of having a bad trip. If you're being honest to yourself, you'd have to admit that all bad trips are nothing else than violent confrontations with fears or unresolved intimate issues, and the DMT trance simply happens to fast.

33

DMT CULTURE

The great body of literature that grew around this mind-blowing mysterious compound has been greatly connected with the grand culture of psychedelics that was born in the sixties. The psychedelic revolution generated an enhancement of perception in a period of liberation from social inhibiting judgments and predetermined forms of thought. It coincided with a fruitful period for human beings when spiritual practices from the East were imported to evolve the pragmatic man of the West. Psychedelic substances played a great role in the rebirth of humanity and the expanding of our collective consciousness such as to receive bright new existential insights.

As such, a lot of the great minds of the period, philosophers, artists and scientists alike engaged in the experimenting with psychotropic substances in clinic environments but also illegally in their own homes, setting the stage for what was to become the study of consciousness.

The books that have been written in that period treat the psychedelic experience in its whole, as it was the new kid on the block, so new that it was hard to discern among its multitude of expressions. Chemists, Shulgin and Hoffman, the discoverers of LSD, were mostly concentrated on studying the visible spectrum of effects and noting each of them along with the respective dosages and chemical interactions.

When it came to the subtle differences in perception and awareness that each psychedelic substance induced, most of the researchers used to talk about the great effect of all of them, too slightly differentiating between their particularities, for it was one grand phenomenon bursting in the human reality all of a sudden, producing such a major shift that none could be something more than the other. As such, most writings about DMT are to be found among the greater presentation of psychedelics in general.

The great prophet of the psychedelic revolution was Timothy Leary, Harvard psychologist and author of the book titled 'High Priest', a precious introduction into the culture of the times, written while he was in and out of jail on reasons concerning exactly the use and promotion of psychedelics. He particularly discusses his own DMT trip as well as other accounts in an article titled 'Programmed communication during experiences with DMT', published in the 'Psychedelic Review'. It is all about breaking the set patterns of perception in order to free your consciousness, as Aldous Huxley praises in his famous novel 'The doors of perception', and as other famous figures as Alan Watts preach in their teachings.

Terence Mckenna, whom we've mentioned quite a few times in this book, was utterly fascinated with DMT. Not as much as he was with psychedelic mushrooms, but still enough to talk for hours on end and write tons of pages about. He was thinking about the 'paradox that DMT is the most powerful yet most harmless of all substances' and being impressed with how 'the human mind can endure that much beauty'.

One of the great figures of our contemporary period discussing DMT is Graham Hancock, who's written and lectured extensively about this compound. His view is that DMT grants us the unique possibility of getting in contact with sentient beings out of our reality, beings that we are otherwise completely unaware of. These entities however know about us and have precious insights that would not only expand our consciousness, but also enrich our material lives and provide extraordinary understandings on how to co-create our common reality within the multiverse.

34

THERAPEUTIC EFFECTS ON ANXIETY & DEPRESSION

As we've talked about, the DMT trip does not directly confront you with the source of your imbalance, rather it takes a more divergent route, presenting you with bewildering settings and characters that don't give you the chance to concentrate on anything else besides that.

In this aspect, it is so much different than Ayahuasca, mushrooms or LSD, substances that are employed in therapy nowadays and that have an obvious action within the psyche apart from the chemical effect within the body. These latter psychedelics induce a psychological trance that is very similar to a therapy session with a psychologist, where you travel inside your own mind, confront and discuss the issues that appear problematic. With DMT, we cannot talk about such action, but nevertheless, this compound has its own means of re-stating the balance within your being.

Recent medical studies inquired a specific strand of DMT, 5-MeO-DMT, commonly found in a lot of plants, but mostly extracted from the venom of the Bufo Alvarius frog. The experiments with this compound on a great number of subjects proved that with only one or two administrations, there was a huge improvement in their overall well-being, with the levels of anxiety and depression decreasing in ways that no other medication or therapy provided before.

The essential advancement that DMT brings forth in comparison with the therapy that engages other psychedelic substances, is the duration of the whole trip. While the magic mushrooms effect, which is now the first in line of research in this matter, takes about nine hours, DMT succeeds in doing at least as good of a job in only half an hour to at most an hour and a half, and this is of major importance for someone who is suffering from acute conditions.

Studies have been undergone regarding the new trend of microdosing, and DMT was administered in microdoses on rats to explore how they react. Indeed, after a little more than a month the rats showed signs of decreased levels of anxiety when inquiring their reactions to fear and past traumas. But there were as well side effects, in that the male rats inexplicably gained weight, whereof the female rats suffered important changes in their neural structures and lost spine density. These studies are only the very first steps in the investigation of DMT though, as this compound is one of the most recent psychedelics to be researched for new medicine.

Nevertheless, if we take just a glimpse on the countless reports of DMT users it might give us a more general and authentic perspective than the precise medical studies. Most of the users confess to an unprecedented improvement on their states of being after consuming DMT, and many of them are approaching this substance specifically in an attempt to heal their anxiety and depression. For all of these, the DMT sessions with full dosage, not microdosing over a longer period, proved to be extremely effective, with this compound being a catalyst for the necessary positive changes that each have to make in their own lives.

DMT helps you find your place in the multiverse, in the multiple parallel realities that coexist with ours, and expand your mind in such a manner that you get to figure out just what's wrong with your current standpoint, and the measures you need to take to rebalance in accordance with the overall reality.

From the background, it reassembles the pieces for you to take on a path of love, peace and lightness, instead of being submerged in heavy past traumas. In this sense, the phenomenon of the ego death is extremely important for it reveals that you are much more than the mental structure impeding your happiness, and helping you go beyond it, in a state where you are able to truly manifest your whole self.

35

BAD TRIPS

It is common knowledge that bad trips on psychedelics, despite their horrific appearance, are actually the most beneficial experiences and present a higher healing potential than the desirable good trips. This is because they are digging out your problems and actually providing solution and relief.

Moreover, you are the one that does all the work so the efficiency of this self-therapy is almost guaranteed, not to mention, the blissful feeling that you most necessarily receive after surviving such an experience, which makes you treasure life in all its complex manifestation.

On DMT, bad trips are a bit different, because it is all concentrated in a very short amount of time and the sensation of being detached from this material reality bypasses the chance of actually connecting the bad trip to some specific problem that you have.

Yes, you may meet unfriendly entities in disrupting environments during your travels, but most of the time the shock is just too big to truly scare you, it's more like watching a very vivid horror movie. More often than not, the bad trip occurs when you haven't paid enough attention to setting this psychotropic experience in a ritualic scenario, that is when you don't show respect towards this worthy substance. Set and setting are essential for all psychedelic endeavors and are the first aspects one has to take care of in the preparation for this journey.

As such, it is preferable to take DMT in a space where you feel most comfortable and calm, in a tidy atmosphere that can ensure your peace of mind, where you don't get interrupted in the middle of the trip. The synergy that DMT induces connects you profoundly with everything around you, so your own home where all is familiar and warm could be a perfect setting.

Nature can also offer a most tranquil environment in which you can immerse safely. On the contrary, if you're not looking for powerful sensations, it wouldn't be advisable to choose an abandoned setting or the club scene. As a matter of fact, most bad trips appear when people use DMT recreationally, ignorant of its huge potential, searching for some glitter when hanging out with their friends and meeting monsters instead.

Spiritual hygiene is the concept that is encompassing all the necessary preparations that you need to do in order to avoid unnecessary unpleasant situations. To summarize its meaning, it is about balancing your state of mind through meditation and setting clear intentions for the voyage you are about to undertake.

The syntagm 'desperate situations require desperate measures' does not go well with the DMT experience, so when you find yourself in an anxiety attack, DMT is not the relief pill for sure. Of course there are a lot of reports from people that were in highly depressive states and took DMT for comfort, receiving enlightening insights which uplifted their grief, but these are exceptions. The point is that whatever the context, you need to be conscious of your actions and assume as your responsibility all that comes towards you.

One other instance when bad trips can occur while doing DMT, like with other psychedelics, is when you don't leave enough time between two different journeys, two different doses. After you've had a psychedelic experience it's advisable to wait a while until you try it again; it's a sign of disrespect towards yourself and towards the trip itself if you rush things, for you didn't offer enough time for the experience to settle, for the understanding to ground inside your being.

Sometimes however, you have bad trips despite your preparation efforts, so you can learn to enjoy them as well. The most important lesson is not to resist the bad trip but accept it, for if you resist it, it will only come at you more forcefully. It may also help to open your eyes and remind yourself that it is just a trip, that you've consumed a psychedelic substance and in a while it will all pass, and you will return to your normal state of being.

Another beneficial piece of advice comes from Terence Mckenna, who, in his turn, borrowed it from the South American shamans, and that is to sing. Whenever a beast like creature that frightens you appears in your scenario, sing to it. When you feel distorted out of recognition, just sing. Whatever comes to mind, sing.

And most of all, do not combine DMT with alcohol or other drugs. This is a recipe for disaster as you will have less control over your thoughts and actions that could lead to poor or dangerous scenarios.

36

THE CURE FOR COLLECTIVE AWARENESS?

We look at our lives irresponsibly in regards to our true nature and we treat the planet in a similar manner as if we are not all connected in the same collective reality. Who are we kidding? We constantly hide our true problems under the carpet, behind the screens of our devices, ignorant to the fact that they don't just disappear and to the harm they are doing to us in the background.

We tend to only choose comfort, and avoid bad trips when it is discomfort and nasty experiences that truly define our reality. What if we chose to confront all these? Maybe it wouldn't be a better world overnight, but it may sure be a more honest attitude.

Of course it takes courage to do this, especially when you feel you are facing the whole of reality by yourself. DMT can show you that you are much larger than you could ever imagine, that you are much more than the social stance that's been imprinted on you, that your role in the whole equation of reality is way more important than the job you are doing or the status you've achieved in your community, that the actual reality is much greater than the most brilliant minds who have defined it. You are important for the simple fact that you exist and that all is interconnected.

DMT might prove to be the most necessary source of wisdom in our fragmented times, the link that can finally dissolve duality and with it the paradox of existence that is making us constantly take sides. This is because it reveals that there are infinite angles and not just two, as humanity has been accustomed to seeing all in black and white.

DMT is finally dissolving this duality, mainly by resolving the conflict between spirituality and science. As we've seen earlier, the beliefs in a greater dimension of reality, as well as in life after death and the facts demonstrated by quantum physics are both reflected in the DMT experience. By transcending duality we may get the ticket to enter another stage in the human evolution, that of a unified reality, and with it, unified humanity.

DMT has the power of awakening the consciousness of the soul inside the individual to the reality that truly is a multiverse of interconnected beings. By this, it awakens the responsibility that each of us has towards their own wellbeing, and towards the wellbeing of our collective environment, which translates in the health of our planet as well as the peace of our collective mental and emotional dimensions. Through such a short glimpse into the complexity of our dynamics, DMT succeeds to truly wake up our spirit and our consciousness.

ALSO BY ALEX GIBBONS

Did you enjoy the book or learn something new? It really helps out small publishers like Alex if you could leave a quick review on Amazon so others in the community can also find the book!

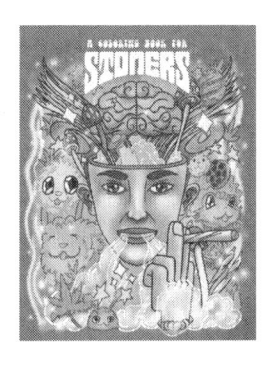

⭐ ⭐ ⭐ ⭐ ⭐

Want to chill and experience the benefits of mindfulness? Want to do something productive while watching random videos on YouTube?

Get this fun stoner themed coloring book to scribble on for your next trip. Search for 'Alex Gibbons Stoner Coloring Book' on Amazon to get yours now!

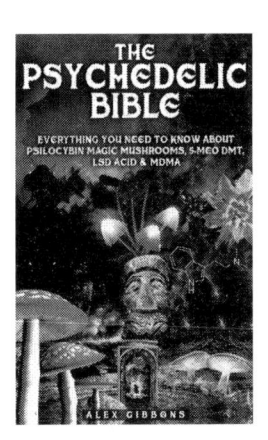

Thinking about taking other magical drugs? Ever wondered what exactly happens when you take them? Want to make sure you don't have a bad trip?

If you want to read more about the history, origins and effects of Magic Mushrooms, LSD/Acid or DMT, search for 'The Psychedelic Bible' on Amazon!

For daily posts on all things Psychedelic, follow us on Instagram @Psychedelic.curiosity

Printed in Poland
by Amazon Fulfillment
Poland Sp. z o.o., Wrocław